Start to empty your fat cells in just 24 hours with...

The
Skinny
Pill™

The top five all-natural, non-prescription supplements that help turn off your fat switch and break your body's food-to-fat cycle

Introducing the companion
"Skinny Food Clock"

A.M. eat fat blocking foods
P.M. eat fat burning foods

Edita Kaye

Here's what they're saying about *The Skinny Pill*...

" I can't believe it! I got my waist back and I'm wearing a belt again..." *Nancy, Florida.*

"My husband lost over 30 pounds, lowered his cholesterol, blood pressure and his prostate tests are back to normal. I reached my goal of 128 lbs and I look and feel terrific..." *Pam, Ohio.*

"Five days into the *Skinny Pill & Skinny Food Clock* I lost 5 lbs—that's a pound a day. Then I went on to lose another 13 lbs in the next 20 days. I have never lost 18 pounds in a month before. My husband says I look great..." *Marg, Washington.*

"I'm a breast cancer survivor and this plan has helped me lose the fat around my middle, gave me more energy, and improved my moods. My doctor says it's great..." *Bobbie, Florida.*

"I have never had this much energy while losing three whole dress sizes before...I love the bedtime snacks and my new shape..." *Wanda, Canada.*

Important Please Read Carefully

The information, ideas, suggestions, and answers to questions in this book are not intended to substitute for the services of a physician. You should only undertake a fat loss, weight loss, and health and wellness modification program in conjunction with the services of a qualified health professional. This book is intended as a reference guide only, not as a manual for self-treatment. If you suspect you have a medical problem or have questions, please talk to your health care professional. All the information here is based on research available at the time of this printing.

Fountain of Youth Group, Inc. 830-13 A1A North, Ponte Vedra Beach, FL 32082
Visit and Shop Online at: www.theskinnypill.com
Call toll free 1-888-7-Skinny or 1-800-870-8087

Printed in the United States of America
First Printing: October 1999
Eighth Printing

Library of Congress Cataloging-in-Publication Data
Kaye, Edita
      The Skinny Pill:/Edita Kaye
      p.   cm.
      ISBN 0-9635150-4-7
      1.   Weight loss. 2. Nutrition.

Meet Edita Kaye

Edita, host of the national PBS television series, *The Fountain of Youth*, guest on H&G TV's *Smart Solutions*, and QVC, is a nutritionist, author and speaker who brings years of experience and commitment to making America healthier and thinner.

Edita wrote *Bone Builders The Complete Lowfat Cookbook Plus Calcium Health Guide.* This wonderful book was a featured alternative of the *Doubleday Book Club* and a selection of the *Literary Guild* and *Crossings Christian Book Clubs. Bone Builders* received many enthusiastic reviews including *The Chicago Sun-Times, The New York Daily News, Redbook* and more...

Next Edita wrote *The Fountain of Youth The Anti-Aging Weight-Loss Program* which was a featured selection of the *Literary Guild* and was excerpted in *The Ladies' Home Journal.* It appeared in *Parade Magazine, First for Women* and many other national publications. This book also went on to inspire a national television series on PBS, and Edita's frequent appearances as the on-air nutritionist for national television shows.

Edita's own story is an inspiration, since she achieved all her success after she turned 50! At 48, alone, broke and abused, the good Lord took her hand and led her out of the dark and into the light. First helping her change her own life, and then helping her change the lives of others.

Funny, witty, motivational, and deeply spiritual, Edita and *The Skinny Pill* have made a real difference in the lives of thousands of Americans, and will make a difference in your life too.

The Skinny Pill

1-800-870-8087

www.theskinnypill.com

Take *The Skinny Pill* Challenge

1. I really try to eat a lowfat diet, but I still can't lose weight.
2. I try to exercise regularly, but nothing much is happening.
3. I'm hungry right after I eat.
4. I crave candy and sugary treats.
5. I gain weight very easily…it seems I just look at a piece of cake and it leaps off the plate and onto my hips.
6. I'm hungry between meals, often.
7. Even if I do manage to lose weight, I gain it all back, and then some.
8. Even if I start to lose weight, I quickly hit a plateau and get stuck.
9. I don't seem to have any energy when I'm on a diet. Everything takes too much effort.
10. I'm so frustrated I could SCREAM. I feel like I'll never lose my fat. Ever.

Scoring: If you answered YES to just one of these statements you and your fat are both excellent candidates for *The Skinny Pill*.

The Skinny Pill Sneak Preview

The Skinny Pill is not a diet.
The Skinny Pill is not about weight loss.
The Skinny Pill is about FAT LOSS.

Within 24 hours...

...your fat cells will begin to empty out.

...your energy levels will soar.

...your cravings will fade.

...your body will begin to regain definition.

...you will begin to lose inches.

...your mood will improve.

...your lean muscle will burn fat more efficiently
and will not be lost while you lose.

...your cholesterol, blood fat, insulin and blood
pressure levels should begin to move
toward healthier ranges.

...your risk for heart disease, stroke, hypertension,
cancer, diabetes, and osteoporosis will be
reduced, improving your life-expectancy.

I know the big question you are asking yourself is, "How is *The Skinny Pill* different from all the other diet books and weight-loss plans I've tried in the past without success?"

Good question. You'll find out as you read. You'll be convinced when you lose. But until then I will tell you this.

The Skinny Pill is like no diet book you have ever read before.

The Skinny Pill is like no weight-loss program you have ever been on before.

Why? Because *The Skinny Pill* isn't about weight loss. It's about FAT LOSS.

The Skinny Pill is about 5 dietary supplements that change your biochemistry from fat attracting to fat rejecting.

The Skinny Pill is about changing your body chemistry in just 24 hours with five miracle nutrients that begin to work on a cellular level to help your body—the best fat-fighting machine ever invented—to dump fat out of your cells and keep it out. Put these 5 supplements together and you have *The Skinny Pill.*

The Skinny Pill is about food. Food that blocks fat. Food that burns fat. It's about eating these fat fighting, skinny foods at certain times during the day. This is the newest, most exciting food plan that gives you 7 meals a day, and organizes your food so that you eat fat blocking foods when the clock says A.M. and fat burning foods when the clock says P.M. This gives you around the clock nutritional fat fighting support.

This is the *Skinny Food Clock.*

Together, the skinny supplements that make up *The Skinny Pill* and the A.M. fat blocking foods and the P.M. fat burning foods that make up *The Skinny Food Clock* are the most innovative, positive and successful fat fighting program in years—a state-of-the-art total fat fighting system based on the most recent studies, both national and international, published by scientific research centers and laboratories specializing in cellular fat reduction research.

The Skinny Pill is about fat fighting supplements.
The Skinny Food Clock is about fat fighting foods.

The Science of Cellular Fat Reduction

In *The Skinny Pill* I have brought you the most exciting and ground-breaking studies from the top research centers in the U.S. and around the world.

Here in *The Skinny Pill* is the latest science that tells us to lose fat and keep it off we need a new weapon in our fat fight. We need more than just another diet. We need more than just another piece of exercise equipment. We need more than a calorie counter. More than boxes of nonfat, low fat, reduced fat—everything. Why?

Because we know diets alone don't work. Exercise alone doesn't work. Nonfat foods alone don't work. We are getting fatter every day. Some estimates say that as many as 70 percent of Americans are too fat. In a room with 10 people— seven are obese—in your office perhaps, your school, your family. We are sinking under an avalanche of fat. Check it out for yourself. Look in a mirror. Look around.

We are losing our fat fight!

But we can win.

The Skinny Pill

What we need is something else. Something new. Something different. Something effective.

> We need a winner. We need a miracle.
> *The Skinny Pill* is our winner!
> *The Skinny Pill* is our miracle!

The Skinny Pill is a scientific and research-based formula designed to work with our own body chemistry—helping it to change from fat loving to fat fighting. In as little as 24 hours, through a combination of five special nutritional supplements—a kind of skinny nutritional cocktail—or "multi-vitamin" for fat—you will begin to empty your fat cells. You will help your body reject new fat while it rapidly burns off stored fat.

The Skinny Pill takes the war on fat deep inside your secret fat pockets, and metabolic processes of your own cells increasing the rate at which you burn fat for energy and helps break the food-to-fat cycle.

The Skinny Pill is a very special formula—a cocktail—a combo of the top five nutritional fat fighting elements designed to attack fat biochemically. This formula helps burn off your existing fat deposits, including the dangerous ones you don't see around your heart and other vital organs and helps block the absorption of new dietary fat. *The Skinny Pill* cocktail does it fast. Efficiently. Hour by hour—from the first 24 hours—even while you are asleep!

With *The Skinny Pill* you get that edge. That head start. That biological boost to finally lose the fat that makes you so unhealthy and so unhappy.

Note: The do-it-yourself *Skinny Pill* formula must consist of the top five fat fighters recommended in this book to get the benefits available. The nutrients are available wherever nutritional supplements are sold, or order Edita's *Skinny Pill* with information listed at the back of the book.

The Skinny Food Clock

A.M. You Eat Fat Blocking Foods
P.M. You Eat Fat Burning Foods

There is more to *The Skinny Pill*. There is *The Skinny Food Clock* that is created to help your body fight fat with every meal. *The Skinny Food Clock* is carefully designed to support your body and *The Skinny Pill* in its fight to rid itself of fat.

The Skinny Food Clock gives you 7 meals a day. Go ahead. Count them.

1. A pre-breakfast
2. Breakfast
3. Morning snack
4. Lunch
5. Afternoon snack
6. Dinner and best of all—
7. A bedtime snack.

Now here is the real nutritional magic of *The Skinny Food Clock.*

You will eat meals that are carefully orchestrated, using real food, to give you major fat blocking nutritional support in the a.m. with satisfying, filling foods loaded with fiber and major fat burning nutritional support in the afternoon, evening and all night long with foods high in protein.

Your A.M. meals will be delicious, filling fat blocking foods high in fiber. Starting with a pre-breakfast!

Your P.M. meals will be delicious fat burning foods, high in protein, including a bedtime snack, that work all through the night, even while you are asleep.

The result? You are just 24 hours away from breaking your own food-to-fat cycle and seeing a skinnier, healthier, you!

Quick Guide To Getting Skinny

The Skinny Pill
Supplement Formula must be a combination of
these top five fat fighting nutrients
Carnitine
Chromium
Citrimax
Chitosan
Citrus Aurantium

The Skinny Food Clock
A.M. eat fat blocking foods. Think fiber.
P.M. eat fat burning foods. Think protein.
Add a fat blocking prebreakfast.
Add a fat burning bedtime snack.

Complete Table of Contents

Sneak Preview

Introduction   *The Skinny Pill* Story

Part One   Eating With The Enemy

Chapter 1   Old Fat Lies & New Skinny Truths

Chapter 2   Getting Skinny: Your Own Personal Fat To Thin Profile

Part Two   *The Skinny Pill*

Chapter 3   *The Skinny Pill* & How It Works

Part Three   *The Skinny Food Clock*

Chapter 9   The Skinny Foods

Part Four   Putting It All Together & Getting Skinny

Chapter 10   Putting It All Together

Part Five Keeping The Skinny Going

Chapter 11   Staying Skinny

Part Six   Cooking Skinny

Oat Bran Balls
Harvest Crisps
Yes, You Can, Strawberry Shortcake
"I'm A Star" Fruit Cobbler
Sweet Trifles

Part Seven   Resources

Introduction

The Skinny Pill Story

It all started with a throbbing headache brought on by a piece of broccoli.

The headache was mine. The broccoli belonged to a small, plump woman with pudgy hands and puffy ankles wearing the standard uniform of the overweight—a loose top over a pair of pants with an elastic waist-band.

The occasion was a meeting of over twelve hundred women in Florida. I was the keynote speaker. The topic was "Eat your way out of middle-age." The response was enthusiastic. We laughed together. We learned together. We bonded over antioxidants. We spent a wonderful hour splashing around in a nutritional fountain of youth.

And now we had all moved into the banquet hall for the requisite post-seminar luncheon.

It wasn't until they served the main course that I even really noticed her, or her friend. We had said our hello's when we first sat down, but there were eight other women at the table and she and I were separated by a vast expanse of water goblets, bread baskets, butter plates, small "goodie" bags bulging with make-up samples and a very pushy centerpiece. We could barely see or hear one another, much less talk.

The Fat Lament

Until the broccoli. There was one of those momentary lulls in the conversation and that's when I heard her say very clearly to her friend sitting on her right, "I don't know what's wrong with me. No matter what I do, I can't lose any weight. No matter how much of this "stuff" I eat, it all ends up on my thighs.

The pre-thigh matter she was glaring at was a piece of broccoli she had speared and was waving on the end of her fork.

Our eyes met. She looked away, embarrassed that an entire table of strangers including the keynote speaker—me—had overheard her fat lament.

It would have ended right there, but another voice chimed in, "I know what you mean…I can't tell you how many diets I've been on that never worked."

Then another voice added, "What about those diets where you lose some weight and gain it all back, plus an extra five pounds, just a few weeks later?"

Suddenly gone were the pleasant, small conversations. The table was now united. Nine women all talking at the same time about their common enemy—fat.

"Did you ever try that combo thigh and ab machine? I used it a couple of times but I'm just too tired when I get home from work to exercise."

"I was going to try some of those prescription diet pills, but my sister's husband's first wife's mother developed some kind of problem when she took them, so I'm really scared."

"I maxed out my VISA card on all that special food I had to buy every week, just to lose a pound or two."

"I'm too embarrassed to go back to all those classes and meetings—my weight is like a yo-yo."

"I'm fine all day—I don't even eat breakfast and I rarely have lunch, but there I am with my face in the fridge, pigging out at midnight."

"I can't eat another nonfat anything—but I'm worried about my kids. They are getting fatter. And I should be the skinny example. But nothing works. I'm just so frustrated."

"I don't know how it happened, but on my forty-seventh birthday my fat moved—now it's around my waist."

"You're lucky. On my forty-seventh birthday my fat not only moved—it multiplied. Now I've got it on my hips *and* around my waist."

And on and on it went. Until my chubby friend, the one with the broccoli, who had by now overcome her initial embarrassment, raised her warm Southern voice over the general weight-loss hubbub and asked, "Edita, what *can* we do to get skinny and stay skinny?"

The Fat Question Needs a Skinny Answer

I was tired. I had just finished a big presentation. I had flown half the night to be with these women. I was hungry. I had a long flight back home. I had the beginnings of a headache. I wanted to be off duty.

So I looked at her and was just about to inhale and make some soothing noise I hoped would satisfy her when I saw her—*really saw her*—for the first time. She was frustrated. Unhappy. In pain.

I looked at the other women at my table in their oversized tops—their size-14 or size-16 suits. The ones with the rolls of fat pushing at the seams of their dresses. The ones sitting stiff and unnatural, bound tight by elasticized full-body girdles. The ones who squirmed trying to get away from panty hose that dug a painful trench around their middle. The ones wearing black—a slimming color. And the ones who had given up altogether and just let it all hang out.

I looked around at the other tables. At the women picking at their lunches. I saw them wave away the potatoes. I watched them scrape the sauce off the chicken before they cut it. I saw full baskets of rolls returned to the kitchen, untouched and unbuttered. I saw desserts scored lightly with forks, but not eaten. I saw over one thousand women—trying—and failing—to be skinny.

My heart went out to her. To all of them. To the overfat husbands and boyfriends they worried about. To the chubby kids they were frightened for. And to me too. Because it wasn't so long ago that I was fat. More than fat—obese. And not a day went by that I wasn't afraid that I would get too tired, too stressed, too old, too hungry, too something—to keep up that fight and that one day I would lose and my fat would win.

I was saved from having to reply by the flickering of lights that signaled the end of lunch and the start of, you guessed it, the fashion show.

Breaking The Food-To-Fat Cycle

But what I didn't know when I left that luncheon, was that I was about to have one of those "eureka" moments that would result in a very happy ending to the sad story of the broccoli that turned to fat—and you are holding it in your hand right now—you are reading it right now.

I didn't know then, as I pushed my way through the post-luncheon crush and into the blazing heat of a Florida summer parking lot, that I was just a few minutes away from finding the answer to that woman's fat question... "What can we do to get skinny and stay skinny?"

I didn't know it then, but I was on the very brink of discovering why, whether she was eating broccoli or donuts—my Florida friend, got fat. Why even when she exercised—she got fat. Why nothing had worked for her long term.

I didn't know it then, but I was about to figure out why everything we eat seems to turn to fat—and I was on the brink of answering that troublesome question once and for all. I was about to discover how we can get skinny and stay that way!

I was on my way to the airport. That faint, slippery little headache was now full-blown pounding surf that surged painfully against my eyelids every time I blinked. But I couldn't get that woman with her piece of broccoli out of my mind.

Why couldn't she lose weight? Why couldn't her husband lose? Why were her kids getting fatter? Why, when she finally managed to lose a few pounds, didn't they stay off? Why did she gain back more than she had lost? Why didn't all those diets work? Why didn't all that exercise get results? Why did more pounds pile on with every passing year? Why? Why?

I was still asking myself those questions when I swung into one of those enormous drug marts to get something for my splitting head before I got on the plane.

There were about fifty different headache remedies. I picked the one closest to me. Bought a bottle of water. And swallowed both right there at the check-out counter.

Five minutes later my headache was miraculously gone! That's when I had my "eureka" moment.

Forget the plane. I turned the car around and headed straight back for that drug store. I rushed up and down the aisles like a woman possessed— and I was. I was possessed of an idea.

There they were. The headache remedies. Shelves and shelves filled with them.

Next aisle over were boxes and bottles and jars filled with heartburn relief.

There was the allergy section.

The cold, cough and flu products got a whole aisle all to themselves.

There were the products for diarrhea and constipation.

Products for a good night's sleep.

Products to stop smoking.

Products to grow hair.

That wasn't all.

Four full aisles were devoted to vitamins and minerals for everything from bone building to stress reduction. There were natural herbs to soothe anxiety, reduce wrinkles, strengthen leg veins, relieve depression. There was even the demon broccoli—powdered and packed into a convenient time-release capsule!

But where was the skinny aisle? Where were the shelves filled with skinny pills? Where was the section devoted to the one product that could help us fight the most dangerous health risk of them all—our own biological stalker—our own individual serial killer—fat?

That's why my broccoli-waving friend couldn't lose her weight or keep it off. All she was using was food—good as far as it went, but it didn't go far enough. All she was using was ordinary exercise—good as far as it went, but it didn't go far enough. And so I asked myself.

What do I do when I have a headache?

I take a pill.

What do I do when I get a cold?

I take a pill.

What do I do when I want strong bones?

I take a pill.

What do I do when I want to protect myself from a heart attack?

I take a pill.

What should I do to get rid of my fat?

I should take a pill.

What should I do to get skinny and stay skinny?

I should take a pill.

For my headache, my cold, my bones, my heart attack prevention I take remedies that work on a cellular level—on a biological level. Remedies that work to fight my headache while I drive. While I think. While I fix dinner or put gas in the car. Remedies that work even while I sleep.

Take A Couple of Skinny Pills and Call Me in the Morning

Is there a skinny pill? Is there something like an "aspirin" for fat? Something like a "multivitamin" to protect me from the negative impact of fat, just as a multivitamin offers protection?

Is there something easy? Fast? Safe? Something I don't need a prescription for? Something natural? Something that works on a biological level? On a cellular level? Is there something that works to make me skinny deep inside my own fat cells, turning them off, dumping them out, shrinking them for good?

Is there something I can take that would alter my fat-loving bio-chemistry, turn off my fat switch and turn on the skinny? Something that would fight my fat and help me get thin and stay thin while I just did the normal kinds of things I do every day? While I ate? Even while I slept?

Is there a skinny pill out there? Turns out there is. Not just a single compound, but an exciting, rich variety of natural supplements that together make up the formula or cocktail I call, *The Skinny Pill.*

The Skinny Pill As Fat Buster

YES we can dump out our own fat. How? With fat fighting nutrients—skinny nutrients—that shovel fat out of our fat cells, transport and dump it into our cellular furnaces where all that stored fat gets burned up and turns into energy. And one of the best of these is carnitine.

YES we can block the absorption of new fat. How? With fat fighting nutrients—skinny nutrients—that absorb four times their own weight in dietary fat. And one of the best of these is chitosan.

YES we can change fat into thin. How? With fat fighting nutrients—skinny nutrients—that wrap dietary fat in a kind of cellular plastic wrap so that it passes harmlessly right through our digestive system, never entering our bloodstream or our fat cells. Again, one of the best is chitosan.

YES we can lower blood fat—cholesterol. How? With fat fighting nutrients—skinny nutrients that bond with fat molecules increasing their overall molecular size and making it impossible for them to pass through the intestinal membrane and into our blood stream. Chitosan, again.

YES we can turn off cravings. How? With fat fighting nutrients—skinny nutrients—that help shut off our "brain tummy" where our cravings for chocolate and potato chips begin. One of the best is citrimax.

YES we can stop the "munchies" and "snack attacks". How? With natural fat fighting nutrients—skinny nutrients—that help regulate our hormonally controlled appestat. Again, here is citrimax.

YES we can "turn on" our own metabolism. How? With fat fighting nutrients—skinny nutrients—that pump up our own body's metabolic rate making it work more efficiently—sort of like getting a biological tune-up or using a better, cleaner grade of biological gasoline. One of the best that nature has provided is citrus aurantium.

YES we can free the lean trapped inside our fat. How? With fat fighting nutrients—skinny nutrients—that help our body retain lean muscle mass, which gives us our youthful shape, definition, the ability to find our waist-line, wear a belt again, and that help break our tragic food-to-fat cycle. One of the most effective of these is chromium.

And here they are, the top five fat fighting nutritional supplements: carnitine, chromium, citrimax, chitosan, and citrus aurantium. Individually these are powerhouses of cellular and biochemical fat fighting ability. Together they are your pathway to fat loss and good health. These are the formula I call *The Skinny Pill*.

The Rest Of *The Skinny Pill* Story

But that's not the whole story here. *The Skinny Pill* is not just about taking a supplement—popping a pill—it's about *The Skinny Food Clock.* A truly remarkable, innovative food plan that works with *The Skinny Pill* to give you even more dramatic, healthy and lasting fat loss results.

Your New *Skinny Food Clock*

When the clock says A. M. you eat meals that are high in fat blocking foods. Foods that have been shown through scientific research to help your body block the absorption of fat. When you think of fat blocking foods, think fiber. You will enjoy a simple, fast and economical menu that starts with a pre-breakfast, then moves on to breakfast, morning snack and lunch.

Then you will switch.

When the clock says P.M. you reach for meals that are high in fat burning foods, think protein. You will start your fat burn with an afternoon snack, go on to a real dinner and finish up your day with a fat burning bedtime snack that will fight your fat while you sleep!

> Seven real meals.
> A.M. foods to block fat.
> P.M. foods to burn fat.
> Too easy.

Here's What Your Skinny Day Looks Like

The Skinny Pill
(either the do-it-yourself formula based on the five top fat fighters or Edita's Skinny Pill)

The Skinny Food Clock

A New Skinny You!

The Day America Won The Fat Fight

We've known we have a weight problem since 1988 when a report by the U.S. Surgeon General estimated that one-fourth of adult Americans were overweight.

But it was only recently that there was a massive, national and very public shift in focus. The fight we now know is not with our weight—but with the real evil—our fat.

For on a warm and sunny June morning in 1998 twenty-six million of us went from just a little chubby—to obese—with one headline. That was the day the *National Heart, Lung and Blood Institute* made national news with its publication of a very scary document—the *Clinical Guidelines on Overweight and Obesity in Adults*. The report pulled no punches. We were found to be fatter than we thought. And fat was killing us.

The report gave us a "quicky" test to check just how fat we were. Forget the bathroom scale. Forget the mirror. Millions of Americans took the test that terrible June morning—the BMI Test—and found that they were suddenly obese. Medically obese!

Forget Overweight Think Overfat

The report on our growing obesity was based on a formula scientists use to measure our body fat. This formula, or test (try it yourself in Chapter 2) is called the Body Mass Index or BMI.

While many of us had heard about the BMI before, we didn't really *get* it. We may have come across it in magazines—right before the "how sexy does your partner think you are" quiz. We may have heard somber docs talking about it as we channel surfed, but we never really grasped the fact that this BMI test would replace the love/hate relationship we've had with our bathroom scales.

The Scale Is Out—The Tape Measure Is In

Well it has. The scale is out. The tape measure is in. Weight now takes a back-seat to fat.

Too much weight scientists now tell us, does not necessarily mean too much fat. Weight alone doesn't tell the whole fat story. After all weight-lifters weigh a great deal. So do body-builders. Wrestlers. Boxers. But their weight is not the result of too much fat—but rather lots of solid muscle.

Big Hair—Long Nails

Weight can also be attributed to other factors. If your scale says you weigh too much it could be because you have big bones. (Some of us really do have big, heavy bones.)

Too much weight could mean you bulked up your muscles—from 98 pound weakling to beach jock—you get the picture.

Too much weight could mean you have big hair. PMS. Long nails. Whatever. Your weight can be attributed to a lot of things—including, but not exclusively—too much fat.

What scientists now want to do is to remove everything that isn't fat from the body weight picture. Leaving—you guessed it—just the fat.

What helped speed up the old "toss the scale" scenario was the fact that experts couldn't agree on a single height-to-weight formula, based on weight scales.

Height-to-Weight Roulette

Back in the fifties, the way you figured out whether you weighed too much, was simple. You looked at a chart that listed your height, your sex, and your ideal weight. You took your finger, found your height and pulled your pinkie across the chart until you found what the 1950s scientists figured was what you should weigh.

Then in the 1980s the numbers were changed—skewed up because scientists then believed that gaining weight as we aged was natural.

In the 1990s the numbers changed again. Now scientists were finding that the lower your weight, the longer your life expectancy might be. So the ideal weight numbers dropped back down.

Up. Down. Back. Forth. The game of height-to-weight roulette left every one dizzy and confused. Who knew what a 5-foot 4-inch woman should weigh? A 5-foot 10-inch man? And if the scientists couldn't get it together, then how could we?

And then came that June morning and the BMI test, and the awful national results.

All of us really understood, perhaps for the first time, that it wasn't really weight, but fat, that counts.

We Are the Fattest People in the World

But the bottom line, so neatly underscored was that Americans—you, me, the woman in front of us at the check-out counter, the bank teller, the clerk at the deli counter, the ad executive, the lawyer, our boss and even our doctor—all of us are too fat. We are the fattest people in the world. And we are getting fatter.

Fat is our special killer. Fat clogs our veins and arteries contributing to our heart attacks and our strokes. Fat stimulates the epidemic growth of our cancers. Fat leads to our massive explosion of diabetes. Our fight is no longer with our weight. Our fight is now with our fat. And this is one fight we have to win...to live!

Fat Stats To Die For

I'm not really big on the scary stats—we all know that fat is killing us in a lot of very unpleasant ways. We know that fat is impacting our health and our lifestyle in every imaginable way from heart attacks and diabetes to dandruff (the more fat you carry, the more likely you have dandruff—it's true, I can't make this stuff up).

But I've found some fat stats that just astounded me, and I think they may astound you, too. Knowing them, may help save your life.

And The Winners In The "Why Are We Getting Fatter?" Category Are...

Did You Know?

The National Center for Health Statistics reports the average American woman today is 5-foot-4-inches tall and weighs 144 pounds.

As if that weren't bad enough, almost 50 percent of us, American women, are a size 14 or higher and by the year 2002 a whopping 42 percent of us will be wearing a size 16 or bigger.

Did You Know?

We don't even have to eat fat to get fat. A new study shows that just tasting or smelling fat is enough to raise levels of triglyceride—a blood fat that is linked to heart disease.

Did You Know?

Even our hospitals are not much help in our fat fight. *The New England Journal of Medicine* reports that a national survey of 57 hospitals found only 7 percent met all federal dietary guidelines— that means that 93 percent of our hospitals serve food that doesn't meet federal dietary guidelines. Thirty-nine percent of all menus for patients with no dietary restrictions contained too much fat and a whopping 81 percent contained too much cholesterol.

Did You Know?

According to the *Institute for Standards Research* in 1942 the average size 8 dress measured 23 ½-inches around the waist and 34 ½-inches around the hips. That's when Bette Davis, Deborah Kerr, Joan Crawford and Susan Hayward strutted their stuff. Today, that same size 8 dress has grown to 27-inches around the waist and 37 ½-inches around the hips. A total of half-a-foot more—all around!

Did You Know?

Time Magazine reports that the average restaurant dinner plate has just gotten 2-inches bigger all around—no doubt to accommodate the huge portions our restaurants are now serving.

And food sizes are getting bigger, too. A pretzel from a New York street vendor or from one of those airport pretzel warmers is equivalent to 5 slices of bread.

And that medium popcorn you just bought at the movies, now contains 16 cups of popcorn!

But here is my all-time favorite, in the "why are we getting fatter" category.

Did You Know?

Handicapped parking fraud rose by 600 percent in some states—indicating that people would rather pay a stiff fine than walk a few extra steps from a more distant parking space to the door of the mall.

Fat Is A Serial Killer

But fat is not funny. Fat is a killer. *The New York Times* reports that 300,000 Americans die each year of obesity. And it isn't pretty. And it isn't cheap. And don't think it can't be you.

75 percent of us are obese. Not pleasantly plump. Not a little chubby. Obese. Here's how fat stalks us and eventually kills us:

Heart Disease
70 percent of the diagnosed cases of cardiovascular disease are related to obesity.

High Blood Pressure
Obesity more than doubles your chances of developing high blood pressure—a major risk factor in stroke.

Breast Cancer
Half of breast cancer cases are diagnosed among obese women. Fat women can't find lumps as quickly, so their breast cancer may go undetected longer. It gets scarier. It seems that fat

may actually activate or trigger cancer cells setting the disease off.

Colon Cancer

Forty-two percent of colon cancer cases are diagnosed among the obese.

Diabetes

Nearly 80 percent of patients with noninsulin-dependent diabetes are obese.

And the list goes on....

And fat is expensive—very expensive. *The Journal, PharmoEconomics* reports that the annual costs of obesity in the United States are estimated at $68 billion.

Thin Thighs First—Then Thin Arteries

A wise person once said, if you keep doing what you've been doing...you'll keep getting the same result. Well, the same result for us is that...

1. We are getting fatter every day.
2. Diets alone don't work.
3. Exercise alone doesn't work.

Welcome to *The Skinny Pill.*
Welcome to *The Skinny Food Clock.*

Here's What's In Store For You

In *Part One* you will begin your journey into the world of The Skinny! You will learn the big fat lies and myths that have kept you a prisoner of your fat and conventional diet programs for years. You will learn some remarkable new truths that will help you shed your fat and move into a healthy, slender life. You will also take three quick, easy tests that will give you an accurate picture of just how fat you are and just how much fat you need to lose.

In *Part Two* you will meet the five top nutritional fat fighters that make up *The Skinny Pill*—that remarkable all-natural, non-prescription supplement formula that will begin to empty your fat cells in just 24 hours, and start you on the wonderful road to a lifetime of slenderness, definition, energy and reduced risk for fat-related life-shortening diseases.

In *Part Three* you experience the eating excitement of *The Skinny Food Clock*. You learn how foods work in harmony and synergy. You learn how eating fat blocking foods when the clock says A. M. and fat burning foods when the clock says P.M.—seven times a day—will help you lose ugly fat, quickly, economically, and easily...without hunger or expense. You will learn how these fat blocking and fat burning foods work around the clock from morning until bedtime and even while you sleep, emptying your fat cells and improving your health.

Part Four is the key section. Here's where you put it all together. This is where your skinny begins and your fat ends.

In *Part Five* you learn how to keep the skinny going. You learn about skinny supporting supplements like calcium, multivitamins and antioxidants, you get a master Skinny shopping list. You also get a 10-minute Skinny Accelerator and loads of choices so you can put your own fat blocking and fat burning meals together.

In *Part Six* you start Cooking Skinny. You make sweet treats, savory treats and you turn America's favorite comfort foods into fat fighters.

In *Part Seven* you get answers to your most frequently asked questions, information for putting your own skinny pill formula together whether you shop your local drug store, health food store, vitamin store or even the internet. And you get all the information you need to order Edita's *Skinny Pill* with an easy web address, an 800 number, a fax number or a plain ordinary vanilla address.

That's it. Welcome to the wonderful world of *The Skinny Pill*!

Ready? Let's get started. Let's get skinny.

Part One

Eating With The Enemy

Chapter 1

Old Fat Lies & New Skinny Truths

Get Naked

That's right. Before we start with the big fat lies and the exciting skinny truths, let's just meet our fat. Let's get to know it. And the fastest way to get to know your fat is to get naked. Get naked and stand in front of a full length mirror. Here's a little tip that comes from my long years of personal experience with fat—you can see lot more of your fat if you stand sideways!

Not a pretty picture is it? But if you're shocked by what you see on the outside, be very, grateful you don't have x-ray vision to see what your fat looks like from the inside. Not fun.

What Exactly Is Fat?

Fat is the leftovers from the food calories our body doesn't use right away for energy. Fat is stored energy. A caloric reserve which our body can draw on in case of famine. Since the only famine most of us experienced was when the pizza order was delivered 15 minutes late—stored energy is something we are not likely to need anytime in the immediate future.

How Does Our Body Turn Food Into Fat?

We eat breakfast. We eat lunch. We throw a few quarters into the vending machine and have a snack. We eat dinner. We have seconds. We pop some corn during commercials. We have a couple of spoonfuls of double-double chocolate chip ice-cream when we put the cat out.

Let's say that's about 2500 calories for the day right there.

Our body takes those calories and gets out all the nutrients it can. Our body uses about 15 percent of the calories we consume, or in this case, 375 calories, for energy to extract food nutrients.

Then it uses about 60 percent of the food calories, in our example, that's 1500 calories, for energy to run our body systems...our heart, our mouth, our brain, and so on...

So we've got 375 calories going for energy to extract nutrients. 1500 calories going for energy to keep living. For a total of 1875 energy calories.

That leaves about 625 extra calories a day.

What happens to those extra calories?

You guessed it.

They turn into fat and our efficient body stores them in case we ever need them again.

If you eat the same way the next day, you've got another 625 extra calories that get stored as fat.

Keep going and in a few days you've got thousands of fat calories.

Now ask yourself. When was the last time you needed thousands of stored fat calories?

Right. Never. And so there they sit. Stored in all the wrong places.

The New Science of Fat

There is a new scientific discipline out there—fat physiology. Its purpose is to study body fat on a biochemical or micro-cellular level. This new discipline is international, a world-wide response to the global epidemic of obesity.

Scientists all over the world are asking themselves the same fat questions we have been asking, and looking for the same skinny answers, we have been looking for, for decades.

What do they ask themselves in their laboratories and their symposia? How about this…

"What is fat?"

"What makes food turn into fat?"

"Is all fat the same fat?"

"Does broccoli turn into fat the same way that a donut turns into fat?"

"How does fat end up in fat cells?"

"How do fat cells get emptied out?"

"Do all calories have equal fat potential?"

"What happens to fat when we restrict calories?"

"What happens to fat when we exercise?"

"Are there foods that actually reduce fat?"

"Can we change our own metabolism and burn up more fat?"

"Is fat genetic…or lifesty e?"

The answers these "fat" scientists are discovering in their labs from New York, to California; from Tokyo to New Delhi; from London to Toronto and beyond to Sydney are exciting, sexy and are turning everything we ever believed about our fat upside down!

Every day new skinny answers to our most troubling fat questions are discovered.

And the implications are profound. We <u>can</u> get skinny. We can <u>stay</u> skinny. And many of these newest findings are right here, in *The Skinny Pill.*

Let's get started.

First let's shatter some very old, very fat, very wrong myths, lies and assumptions. Ready?

Eat Less, Weigh Less

You've probably already had lots of personal experience with this one. You need to lose. So what do you do? You stop eating. You skip breakfast. You have a cup of black coffee for lunch—maybe even a cigarette. Dinner rolls around and you pick at a salad. Then you spend the night chewing your fingernails and trying not to think about food.

The first couple of days you lose about two or three pounds—mostly because you are running to the bathroom once every forty minutes to empty your bladder.

The next couple of days you lose another pound.

And then, NOTHING!

You are stuck.

You skip dinner.

Still NOTHING!

You add a 30-minute walk to your day.

NOTHING!

You dust off your exercise bike.

Oh, no. Now you have GAINED a pound!

Disgusted. You go out for pizza and beer.

Your diet is shot...again.

How many times have you gone through this same cycle asking yourself, "Why is it that the less I eat, the less I lose?"

Here is one of the biggest and most stubborn of all the big fat myths we have come to believe. In fact the opposite will give you a better outcome...Eat More—Lose More.

Here's why.

When you eat fewer than 1200 calories a day, your body thinks your world is out of food. It believes all the fast-food restaurants have closed. The supermarkets are empty. And the only thing in your fridge is a light bulb.

And so, because your body needs between 1200 and 1800 energy calories a day to keep your heart beating, your lungs breathing, your eyes blinking and your brain thinking—it slows down your metabolic rate in order to conserve energy calories. Your body figures that since no new energy calories are coming in, it is going to have to depend on stored energy calories—fat.

The result? You become stuck. Frustrated. And give up.

The New Skinny Truth: Eat More Weigh Less

By keeping your body fueled with 1200 to 1800 calories a day, you will keep your fat burning engine running smoothly.

To increase your fat loss you can then stimulate your own body's ability to burn fat with natural fat burning supplements such as the ones found in *The Skinny Pill* formula.

You can boost your fat burn even more with "hot calorie" foods. These are foods that cause your body to work extra hard and use up extra energy to extract their nutrients and digest them. Proteins, such as the ones in *The Skinny Food Clock,* which you will be eating when the clock says P.M. will keep your body burning fat fuel all afternoon, evening and into the night while you sleep.

The Lowfat Myth: Eat Less Fat, Be Less Fat.

Let's clear something up right away. Once and for all.

You aren't getting fatter because you are eating too much fat.

No. In fact you are eating less fat than ever.

And I *know* you are eating less fat.

How do I know this?

Because the *Department of Agriculture* tells me so. It reports that in 1977 fat comprised 40 percent of our daily diet. In 1991 fat consumption went down to 34 percent of our daily diet. And by 1996 fat consumption went down again, and fat comprised only 33 percent of our total calories.

All in all our total fat consumption has dropped by 17.5 percent BUT our obesity has increased by 25 percent.

Go figure.

We aren't getting fatter from fat.

The Skinny Truth

We are getting fatter from bigger portions. Experts believe that when we eat foods that are marked nonfat, low fat, reduced fat we take it to mean that we can eat more, without penalty.

The truth is, while the fat content of these foods may be reduced, the calorie count often is exactly the same.

Check it out for yourself. Look at a jar of reduced fat peanut butter. Now look at a jar of regular peanut butter. Even though one has less fat, they both have the same number of calories.

That's why we are eating less fat but still getting fatter.

Here's where The Skinny Pill provides a complete turn-around in thinking and results in a rapid loss of fat. Stop taking fat out of food—as in no fat, lowfat, reduced fat—and start putting in biochemical fat fighters such as the 5 mega skinny supplements in *The Skinny Pill.* What a concept!

The 30% Big Fat Myth

Here's another shocker. This one has to do with the magic number 30. We've all heard the warning hundreds of times. Don't eat more than 30 percent of your daily calories as fat. If you can keep your daily fat intake to 30 percent of your total daily calories your health will improve.
But will it? Did it?

The 30% Skinny Truth

In 1995 the *National Heart and Lung Institute* in London released a shocking study during the *First International Conference on Fats and Oils and Human Disease.* They reported that two large clinical trials, conducted over a span of twenty years—that's two decades of food and fat—failed to demonstrate that keeping fat calories at 30 percent of our daily diet has a positive effect on our health.

Experts shocked the nutritional world by admitting that reducing our daily intake of fat calories to 30 percent doesn't work.

We are fatter than ever.

And still we continue to buy almost $30 billion of fat-reduced food including $15 billion worth of fat-challenged snack foods—a category that didn't even exist before 1992.

The Fat Cell: Fact & Fiction

"It's not me...it's my female fat cell."

Good one.

First of all the fat cell was first one of the skinniest cells in our body. That's right.

It's true we have between 30 and 50 billion fat cells—or adipose cells in our body. Each one of those cells has the capacity to store 0.5 micrograms of fat—that's a total of about 33 pounds!

But these cells were once the skinniest cells in our body.

Picture a deflated balloon. It's flat. It's thin. It's skinny. Well that is a fat cell.

Now picture that balloon filled with hot air. It's fat. It's round. It's big. Well that's also a fat cell.

In fact fat cells and balloons have a lot in common, structurally speaking. What we call a fat cell is simply a cell with a large empty storage space in the middle—like a balloon. It stays flat and skinny until we fill it with fat.

The Making Of A Fat Cell

Fat cells start off empty. As we continue to eat more food than we need these cells begin to fill up with fat—a process called hypertrophy.

If we run out of storage space in the first batch of fat cells, our body obliges us by creating more—a process called hyperplasia.

So if you keep eating. Adding fat. Making more fat cells, you could end up with up to 100 billion fat cells all ready and waiting for you to fill them up with fat. You definitely want to avoid making any new fat cells. It is possible to empty out the stored fat in your fat cells—flattening them—like a balloon is flattened again once you let the air out. But it isn't possible to make fat cells themselves disappear.

Last Fat In—First Fat Out

When fat cells fill up—we gain. When fat cells empty out—we lose.

Which fat cells fill up first and in what order is thought to be regulated by our gender, our age, our race and genetics. But in watching the in-and-out flow of fat, scientists have made a remarkable discovery.

The last cells to fill up with fat when you gain, are the first ones to empty out when you start to lose.

If you gained and gained and finally your waist disappeared—you'll probably first be able to wear a belt again, when you start to lose. If you finally developed saddlebags—you'll first get your great thighs back when you start to lose. If you finally noticed your bust bursting out of your bra— you'll first go down a cup size when you lose.

The Great "All Fat Is The Same," Myth

All fat is not the same. There are two kinds.

Vanilla Fat and Strawberry Fat

Most of our fat is a yellowish-white color. This is the fat that sits just under the skin, around our hips, our thighs, our bellies, our buttocks...let's call this fat, vanilla.

But not all our fat is vanilla. Extending across our backs, from arm pit to arm pit, and wrapped snuggly around our hearts, kidneys, livers, and other vital organs is a blanket of thick, brownish-pink fat, filled blood vessels. Let's call this fat, strawberry.

Strawberry fat has a very special function. It protects our vital organs from bumps and keeps them warm. Like that pink attic insulation. It makes no difference whether you live in Alaska or Hawaii—you've got insulation—and it's strawberry fat.

Strawberry fat is also critical in helping us lose fat. That's right. You see, this brownish-pink organ fat takes a long time to burn off. But when it starts to burn, it burns hotter, uses more energy, goes through more fat calories, than our plain vanilla fat. Skinny supplements, like the ones in *The Skinny Pill* formula, that can help bring the burn to our strawberry fat can help us lose more fat, faster.

The Real Estate of Fat

There is a saying in real estate...location, location, location. Well, location is critical in our personal fat geography as well.

Fat is much more dangerous to our overall health when it wraps itself around our middle, giving us a distinctive apple shape.

Historically, this gut or "beer belly" was a guy-thing. Not any longer. As more and more women reach fifty-one—the average age of menopause—they also find that among the more unpleasant and dangerous side-effects is a shift in female fat from the hips and buttocks to the waist. Women go from a classic pear shape to a pear and apple shape—or a fat fruit cocktail!

But all kidding aside. These middle-body fat cells are believed to more readily dump their load

71

of fat into key blood vessels, too close to the heart, increasing our risk for heart disease, whether we are male or female. Fat is bad enough as a health risk. Gut fat is a major risk factor for heart disease, currently the number one killer of both sexes.

Fat Is Hereditary

Yes. And no. Thousands and thousands of years ago, when we humans were evolving, fat storage was important to make sure we didn't starve between meals. And meals were few and far between. Back then our dinner often ran faster than we did. Fat was so important to our survival not only as individual humans, but as a species, that researchers today speculate we may be genetically programmed to crave the taste of fat—so that we keep eating it to never run out.

Women, entrusted biologically with promulgating the species, needed more fat for energy than men. We needed it, especially around our hips to protect our wombs and to keep the fetus we carried warm and insulated. We needed it around our breasts to nurse our infants. And so biology gave females more fat and a greater craving for fat. That explains why our female fat makes up a generous 15 to 30 percent of our total body mass.

For men, who got programmed into running around and chasing down dinner, the percentage is a little lower. Male fat makes up between 12 and 25 percent of men's total body mass.

The All Fat Is Bad Myth

Wrong. Fat isn't all bad. It has a very important good side. The truth is we need a certain amount of fat to transport vital fat soluble vitamins to our cells. Vitamins A, E, K, and D are critical antioxidants and offer real biological protection against disease. Without fat they would have no cellular transport.

We also need a certain amount of fat for insulation to keep us and our vital organs warm and protected.

The Metabolism Myth

"Fatties" have slower metabolisms than "Skinnies". This is probably my all-time favorite big fat lie. I've used it myself. I can still hear myself whining that the reason I'm fat is because I've got a slower metabolism than all those "skinnies" out there.

Wrong. Wrong. Wrong.

In fact just the opposite is true.

The fatter you are, the faster your metabolism.

The thinner you are, the slower your metabolism.

Now I'm going to prove it to you with the help of some very exciting new science.

First of all write down your lowest adult weight. You remember. That's the weight you were when you wore that size 10 outfit, the one hanging at the back of your closet for ten years just in case you get down to a size 10 again. How much did you weigh back then? 110? 117? 125? Whatever it was, write it down

Now write down your highest adult weight. That's right. You remember when that was—

perhaps it's now—now when you are into "big shirts," and elastic waistbands on your pants. Now, when you've started to tease your hair again so you don't look like you have this tiny little head on this huge body. Go ahead. Nobody is watching. Write down your highest adult weight.

Resting Metabolic Rate or RMR To Its Friends

Most of the calories we burn up every day are burned to provide us with the energy we need to keep our body alive and functioning—to keep our heart beating—our brain thinking—our hair growing—our kidneys flushing—our bowels moving—our lungs breathing. All that work is going on all the time, day and night, whether we are asleep or awake. Scientists call this ongoing body work our resting metabolic rate or RMR. This RMR uses up between 60 and 70 percent of our total calories.

The RMR is important in the new fat science.

What's Your Personal RMR?

Want to know how many calories you burn up every day, just living? Here's the simple formula. Just get out your calculator.

$$\frac{\text{Your weight in pounds x 24 (hours in a day)}}{2.2 \text{ (kilograms)}}$$

Your weight in pounds divided by 2.2 (kilograms) and multiplied by 24 (the hours in a day) equals your personal Resting Metabolic Rate. This gives you the number of calories your body burns up every 24 hours just keeping you alive.

Got it?

Now let me show you how the fatter you are, the more calories your body actually burns.

Stay with me.

Now, take your lowest adult weight. Let's say it was 110. Here's how the math works out.
$110 \div 2.2 \times 24 = 1200$

Your body used up 1200 calories when you weighed 110 pounds every single day just to keep your systems going.

Now take your highest adult weight. Let's say it was 169. Here's how the math works out.
$169 \div 2.2 \times 24 = 1843$

Your body used up 1843 calories when you weighed 169 pounds every single day just to keep your systems going.

Your RMR used more calories when you were fatter than when you were thinner! The fatter you are, the more calories your body burns!

Chapter 2

Getting Skinny
Your Personal Fat-To-Thin Profile

How fat are you?

If you can't remember the last time you wore a top tucked neatly into your pants, you know you are too fat.

If you can't look down and see your knees because they are hidden by a mound of tummy, you know you are too fat.

If you have to "suck it in" every time you struggle into your freshly washed jeans or skin your fingers and break your nails, trying to zip them up, you know you are too fat.

Or it could be that your blood pressure is up. Your pulse is too fast. Your cholesterol levels are out of whack. Perhaps you have just been told you have diabetes. It could be that you can't get up in the morning without aches and pains and the stiff, shuffling of someone much older than you. It could be that every meal gives you heartburn or indigestion, or both. It could also be that you feel depressed, disgusted and hopeless.

If that's you, you already know you are too fat. What you might not know is just how "too fat" you are. Don't worry. *The Skinny Pill* is going to help you lose that fat. But first let's just find out how much fat you are really carrying around.

How Much Of You Is Fat?

The bathroom scale has been a permanent fixture in our lives since our first check-up. We gain by it. We lose by it. Up till now we've lived by it. Guess what? The scale is out. Why? Because it measures more than just your fat. It measures your total weight, including your bones, muscles, organs, your body water AND your fat.

That's not what we want to measure. We are only interested in how much body fat we have and how much body fat we need to lose to get into the healthy range. Today, medical science tells us that our good health, longevity and vitality are not only the result of the number of total pounds on our bodies, but the number of fat pounds.

Are You Steak or Bacon?

Try this. Think of yourself as 16 ounces of meat. You could be 16 ounces of steak—a juicy, lean sirloin—or you could be 16 ounces of bacon, streaked with wide stripes of fat. Both the steak and the bacon weigh exactly the same—16 ounces or one pound. But the pound of steak is 41 percent fat. While the pound of bacon is 77 percent fat— almost twice as much. Do you want to be steak? More lean muscle than fat? Or do you want to be bacon? More body fat than body lean.

Fat—Overfat—Obese: How Fat Is Fat?

The prestigious *World Health Organization*, the *National Institutes of Health*, *The American Health Foundation*, and dozens of other national and international medical and scientific groups now urge us to focus on our fat—the amount we have and where we carry it. The percentage of our total body mass that is fat and where that fat is stored, are the critical measures of how healthy we are, how long we'll live, and how well we will look and feel.

Where is the fat vs. lean line? Scientists and medical experts have now drawn that line at a total fat content of 16 to 19 percent body fat for men and 22 to 25 percent body fat for women. This is now the ideal and healthy amount of fat to carry. Deviate from that scientifically established range by more than 5 percent you are considered overfat. Move out of that range by more than 25 percent (for men) or 35 percent (for women) and you become medically obese.

Where do you and your fat fit? Let's find out.

The Three Fat Tests

Here's What You'll Need

A fabric tape measure
A calculator
A bathroom scale
A pencil or pen
A pad of paper
A sense of humor

1. The Body Mass Index or BMI Test

This test uses a precise mathematical formula to measure just how much of you is fat. This measure of fatness is based on both your height and your weight. Scientists have determined that the total amount of fat you carry is a critical indicator—not necessarily how many pounds you weigh. (Don't toss that bathroom scale yet, you'll need it here.) Ready? Begin.

a) Step on your scale and make a note of your weight.

b) Multiply your weight by 700.

c) Divide this number by your height in inches.

d) Divide that number by your height in inches once again.

e) The number you get is your BMI.

How do you score?

Dangerously thin	15
Optimum	21
Overfat	25
Obese	30
Dangerously obese	35

My BMI is: _____

2. The Fruit Test

Fat researchers now believe that <u>where</u> your fat is located on your body is as important as how much of it you have. I call this one the Fruit Test. But it is also called the Apple or Pear Fat Test or by its more scientific name, the Waist-to-Hip Ratio Test.

Women typically collect fat (as we already know) in our hips, buttocks and thighs giving us a distinctive "pear" shape.

Men typically collect fat around their bellies giving them more of a rounded "apple" shape. This apple shape puts men at a greater risk for obesity-related diseases and has been linked to shorter life expectancy.

After menopause, many women not only collect fat in their hips, buttocks and thighs, but also around their middle—putting post-menopausal women at the same increased risk as overfat men.

Ready? Begin.

a)   Take the fabric tape measure and measure your waist at its narrowest point. Can't find your narrowest point? Measure around the level of your belly button.

b)   Now measure your hips at their widest point. That shouldn't be too hard to figure out.

c)   Divide the waist number by the hip number. That gives you your Apple or Pear result or your Waist-to-Hip Ratio.

Scoring:

Women

Ratios below 0.8 are in the acceptable zone.
Ratios higher than 0.8 are over fat and at risk.

Men

Ratios below 1.0 are in the acceptable zone.
Ratios higher than 1.0 are over fat and at risk.

My Apple or Pear Ratio is: _____

3. Fat Waist Test

Canadian obesity researchers have recently developed a new test which is proving to be very simple and very accurate. All you need is a tape measure and a waist. Simply take your waist measurement at belly button level.

Men

Waist 40 inches or more	Lose fat
Waist 37 to 39 inches	Don't add fat
Waist 36 ½ inches or less	O.K. zone

Women

Waist 36 inches or more	Lose fat
Waist 31 ½ to 35 ½	Don't add fat
Waist 31 inches or less	O.K. zone

My waist measurement is: _____

These three tests will confirm what you already know. Your health. Your looks. Your life may depend on how much of your fat you can now lose and keep off.

Bonus Measurements Test

Before you begin *The Skinny Pill* and *The Skinny Food Clock* write down your measurements. Wait 5 days and take them again. And take them again after your first month. You should be very pleasantly surprised. In fact, many people get a hint even before they take their measurements after being on *The Skinny Pill*—their clothes hang loose!

Measurements	Start	5-Days	30-Days
Weight			
Waist			
Chest			
Hips			
Upper Thigh, Left			
Upper Thigh, Right			
Calf, Left			
Calf, Right			
Upper Arm, Left			
Upper Arm, Right			

Part Two

The Skinny Pill

Chapter 3

The Skinny Pill and How It Works

The New World Of Biochemical Fat Fighters

Think of a multivitamin. What do you get? You get some vitamins. What do they do? Well, different vitamins do different things. And many of them do more than one thing.

Take vitamin C for example. It prevents you from getting scurvy. It helps keep your skin youthful. It is a powerful antioxidant that floats around in the warm soup between your cells.

Now take vitamin E. It protects the fatty parts of your cells from attacks by free radicals. It is the "sex" vitamin enhancing potency. It protects you from certain forms of cancer.

What else do you have in that multiple vitamin? Well, you probably have some minerals. You might have selenium, a wonderful antioxidant mineral. You might have calcium that helps keeps your bones strong and saves you from osteoporosis and possibly colon cancer. You've probably got some iron, some B vitamins...you get the idea. One multiple vitamin. Lots of nutrients. Lots of health in lots of different biochemical ways.

How long does it take your multiple vitamin to start drenching your cells with goodness and health? An hour? Two hours? It starts working as soon as you swallow it. Right? That's the same concept behind *The Skinny Pill.*

Think "Multivitamin"—Think *The Skinny Pill*

Think of *The Skinny Pill* as a kind of "multivitamin" for skinny—a kind of fat fighting multiple vitamin. The formula contains not one, not two, not three—but five major nutrients that attack fat in different ways. Breaking it down. Flushing it out. Reducing your cravings for it. And more. These fat fighters offer cellular protection in addition to their strong fat reducing function.

Individually these skinny nutrients work with your own body to help block new fat from being absorbed. They can crank up your fat burning furnace to speed the chemical process of turning fat into energy calories and reversing the calories into fat formula. These nutrients can create even more fat fighting power by helping preserve and in some cases, even increase, lean muscle mass. They can help normalize your appestat so your hunger and cravings don't rage out of control. That's what they can do individually.

Taken together, in combination, they act synergistically to become a powerful biological force that can begin to biologically change your body chemistry from fat storing to fat shedding in twenty-four hours or less. They can help you break the killer food-to-fat cycle.

Rapid Cellular Delivery

How fast does *The Skinny Pill* work? As soon as you swallow it...as soon as it enters your system. That's how fast it starts turning on The Skinny and turning off, the fat.

Chapter 4

Carnitine: The Fat Garbage Truck

It's very early Saturday morning. You'd rather be sleeping, but instead, you're packing up a load of boxes filled with all the junk that's taken over your life. That's why on this beautiful Saturday morning you're stuffing boxes, dragging them out to the curb for the garbage truck and the trip to the incinerator.

It's twelve hours later—Saturday night. You've got your feet up and you're looking around. Wow! Check out all the space around you. Suddenly you've got lots of room. Your closets are empty. Your hallways are uncluttered. There even seems to be more air to breathe. And all thanks to a garbage truck and an incinerator.

That's pretty much the same thing l-carnitine does deep inside the energy field of every single one of your cells. It's an intracellular garbage truck picking up fat from its old storage compartments--you know, the ones around your thighs, your hips, your belly, under your upper arms and even around your heart--and moving it out, into cell furnaces, or little cell incinerators called mitochondria, where it's burned up as fuel for energy. The result? Less fat. More energy.

The Supernutrient L'Carnitine

L'carnitine is a very unique supernutrient. Not quite an amino acid, and not quite a vitamin. It's a nutritional hybrid with a very crucial job in fighting fat.

L'Carnitine At Work

L'carnitine's job description is to move fatty acids (fondly known to its friends as fat globs) from their storage bins in fat cells, through delicate cell membranes, and dump them into mitochondria—internal cellular furnaces.

Mitochondria are power rods deep inside each one of our cells. These mitochondria are like microscopic furnaces burning up fat and turning food into 90 percent of all body energy. The more active your body is, the more mitochondria you have and the more energy they produce. The result? We have more energy and less fat.

L'carnitine, then, helps to burn off stored fat. That in itself is pretty remarkable.

But that's not all it does. There's more. While it burns this fat, it also increases your energy levels. This in turn cranks up cellular fat burning ability so that the fat burning circle widens—even as you get thinner and more energized.

Appetite Suppressant

Wait, there's still more. Studies show that l'carnitine may reduce feelings of hunger and food cravings that sabotage so many of our fat loss attempts.

And, like so many nutrients, l'carnitine does even more to keep us healthy and vigorous, than just move and burn fat. Promising research shows that l'carnitine…

> …**promotes** normal growth and development.
>
> …**boosts** energy and endurance during exercise, for a better workout.
>
> …**assists** our hearts to use existing oxygen more efficiently.
>
> …**lowers** high blood cholesterol levels keeping our blood vessels clear and healthy.
>
> …**raises** the levels of "good cholesterol" (HGH).
>
> …**increases** our physical stamina.
>
> …**helps** our body build muscle which in turns helps burn more fat and keep us lean.
>
> …**protects** us from developing diabetes.
>
> …**reduces** our risk of developing liver and kidney disease.
>
> …**enhances** the effectiveness of sperm.
>
> …**fights** against depression.

…**sharpens** our mental acuity, optimizes our brain energy and may be a major nutritional weapon in our war on Alzheimer's and our most valuable brain longevity nutrient.

Take The L'Carnitine Challenge

1. I lack energy for all the things I want to do.
2. I want to lose some weight.
3. I want to improve my heart health.
4. I want to strengthen my immune system.
5. I'm a vegetarian.
6. I'm under a lot of stress and pressure.
7. I keep fighting chronic health problems.
8. I'm in a high risk group for cancer.
9. I'm in a high risk group for diabetes.
10. I want and need maximum daily performance at work and at play.

Score: If you answered YES to even one of these points you are an excellent candidate for l'carnitine cellular therapy.

Your Perfect Carnitine Fat-Burning Day

If you are not a vegetarian you will get about 50 mg of carnitine from the foods you eat. Here is one good reason for digging into that steak...red meat is the best dietary source of carnitine. Go ahead, put lamb chops back into your diet and mutton, and steak. But don't forget to add chicken and turkey, also good sources. And third on the dietary carnitine hit parade are dairy foods.

Vegetarians don't despair. Tempeh (a soy product) and avocado are also good sources of dietary carnitine.

Optimal Daily Dose

250 to 500 mg
Always take with 8 ounces of water.
Some experts recommend up to 1000 mg of carnitine a day taken in two divided doses.

NOTE: Look for l'carnitine—the form that is biologically active and is the same natural form as found in animal or plant tissue.

Chapter 5

Chromium: The Fat Microwave

Solving The "Eat Less—Lose Less" Puzzle

Is this you? There you sit, for the fourth day straight, in front of your dinner—a microscopic piece of chicken, a lettuce leaf and a glass of water. Not great, but at least it beats your lunch which was two gulps of a canned protein drink which the label optimistically dubbed a "nutritious meal substitute shake." It might have been nutritious, but it was no meal substitute and didn't even come close to resembling a shake. Then again it could have been worse. It could have been a repeat of your breakfast for the past four days since your diet began—just black coffee.

Let's face it. You're starving. You obsess about food all the time. You have zero energy. You're cranky and irritable. Your cravings are torture. You've run out of scratch pads to add up your pathetic daily allotment of 550 calories. You've run out of diet soda. You've run out of sympathetic friends.

But you still cling to the only thing you do have left, hope. Hope that tomorrow, on day five of this self-imposed deprivation you call a crash diet, your bathroom scale will reward you. By the miracle of starvation you will have lost five pounds, six pounds, maybe even ten pounds. You hold fast to the hope that your fashionably slim body will just slip into that slinky new outfit. That your tummy will have disappeared. That your midriff will be bikini flat. That your bust won't spill out over your bra cups. That even your ankles will be slender and your feet won't puff around your sandal straps.

And then you step on the devil scale. Nothing. Not a single ounce. You step on. You step off. You move the scale hoping to find a skinnier piece of bathroom tile. That's even worse. Now the scale shows you've gained half-a-pound!

Despair, frustration and yes, even rage, hurl you toward the fridge where you stand stuffing down four days worth of all the food you had denied yourself, and then some...your diet dreams shattered once again.

What happened? You've just become another victim of the Eat Less—Lose Less Fat Puzzle. Enter the solution to the Eat Less—Lose Less Puzzle—Chromium. Stay tuned.

The Yo-Yo Diet Syndrome

How about this. Is this you? You've finally done it. It only took about 100 baggies of raw carrots, 12 weekly meetings and weigh-in sessions, over a thousand dollars of pre-packaged diet foods that strained your VISA card to the max, and 90 nights of crawling into bed at six o'clock, trying to fall asleep before you got attacked by the midnight munchies.

Here it is, finally, day 91 of your diet. You stuck to it this time and you have been rewarded. You've lost fifteen pounds! You congratulate yourself. You rush out and buy that new outfit in the smaller size. You suddenly love looking at yourself in the dressing room mirror. Your friends are full of admiration—and envy. You go out to celebrate. You know the rest. A couple of weeks later not only have you gained back the fifteen pounds you lost, but a bonus of an extra five pounds! What happened? You've just become another victim of the Yo-Yo Diet Syndrome.

Enter chromium picolinate, the solution to Yo-Yo Diet Syndrome. and one of the most exciting and powerful nutritional fat fighters available. Stay tuned.

Take The Chromium Challenge

1. The less I eat, the less I lose.
2. Even when I do lose weight I gain it all back, and a few extra pounds besides.
3. My doctor says my cholesterol level is too high.
4. I'm in a high risk group for diabetes.
5. I suffer from sweet cravings.
6. My energy really slumps in the afternoon.
7. I suffer from mood swings.
8. My memory isn't as good as it should be.
9. I am between the ages of 45 and 55.
10.I am concerned about developing osteoporosis.

11.There is a history of heart disease in my family.
12.I suffer from arthritis.
13.I have been diagnosed with hypertension.
14.I'm under a lot of stress every day.
15.I eat a lot of processed foods and drink a lot of canned sodas.

Scoring: If you answered YES to even one of the above points, you are in the chromium deprivation zone. But you're not alone. About 90 percent of us don't get enough of this skinny supplement, especially as we get older.

So, What Is Chromium, Anyway?

Chromium is what scientists call an essential trace element or an essential trace mineral. It's a mineral our body needs every single day but can't produce so we have to get it from dietary sources and supplements. Chromium is……

…a thermogenic agent, reducing body fat without traditional dieting or exercise. Wow!

…an insulin cofactor, helping this hormone regulate sugar and blood fat more efficiently. Wow, again!

What Makes It Such A Great Fat Fighter?

For such a micro miracle, chromium is all over the place fighting fat in some of the most ingenious ways nature ever invented.

1. Boosts Fat Loss Without Diet Or Exercise

Remember the eat less—lose less fat puzzle? Remember the yo-yo diet syndrome? The reason both these frustrating results happen is that when we diet to lose weight we lose a combination of about 70% fat and 30% (some reports put this as high as 50%) lean muscle. Short term this gives us a false sense of success.

Because the lean muscle that we lose along with the fat slows down our metabolism. When that happens we slow down the rate at which we burn off remaining fat and our fat loss also slows down to a trickle—not pounds of fat coming off any more—just pathetic little ounces.

The less muscle we have the less fat we burn and the less fat we lose. That's what happens in round one. That's the eat less—weigh less problem.

In round two of our diet fight we begin to gain back the weight. Only what we gain back is 110% fat and 30% lean muscle. Because our body is not so dumb on a cellular level. Once we start eating normally again, adding calories to our diet, our body hoards those calories in case we decided to diet and deprive it again. This time, our body chemistry makes more fat and less muscle. We are worse off than before we started. That's why we not only often gain back our original fat, but an extra few pounds as well, pounds that should have been new muscle. We keep losing precious lean muscle tissue with every round of fat loss. Long term, it sabotages every single ounce we want to keep off.

Why? Because one of the ways to lose fat is to burn more of it off. And one of the best ways our body has of burning off fat—is through muscle. The less muscle tissue we have, the less fat we burn, the less weight we lose. That's the yo-yo syndrome.

Both the eat less—lose less and the yo-yo diet syndrome are about muscle, as well as fat.

That's why chromium is such a dream player on our skinny team. It helps us burn fat without losing muscle—even while we sleep. The result? More fat loss. Longer-lasting fat loss. YES!

A Bonus Benefit

All that extra muscle we don't lose. Guess what it does? Give us definition so that we begin to look lean as we get lean.

---

2. Mitigates the *Garden of Eden Effect*

You eat on the run. Stop at the drive-thru window more than once a week. You snack from the vending machine. You order in most nights. You take out on the nights you don't order in. Dinner comes out of a box, a package, a can.

If this is you, you are suffering from what scientists have termed the Garden of Eden effect— a diet that consists of virtually all processed foods with few whole foods. Eating this way puts you on the nutritional fast track to being a blimp— chromium helps mitigate these fast food negatives.

3. Improves Your Thyroid Performance

Remember blaming your weight gain on your thyroid? And remember how all your skinny friends rolled their eyes and kept urging you to stop your secret binging—even as you were starving yourself? Well, you were the one who was right. At least partly right. Your thyroid hormones do regulate your body's basal metabolic rate— your couch potato rate—the calories you burn doing absolutely nothing but breathing and digesting. Chromium improves the status of your thyroid and helps to boost your basic metabolism so that more body fat is burned.

4. Regulates *The Insulin Fat Burning Cascade*

Insulin is a doorkeeper hormone. It's our hormonal cop, directing nutritional traffic through our highway of blood vessels and into each one of our 70 trillion cells. And like most highways, our blood highway is clogged with traffic, including sugar and fat. Insulin's job is to move that sugar and blood fat out of the traffic stream and into working cells for energy. If the cells are working properly, they open up and just enough fat is deposited to provide body energy and insulation.

But nothing works perfectly all the time. Sometimes our cells become insulin resistant and put up insulin barriers. What happens? If insulin can't cope with the flow of blood fat and sugar, it simply moves these off the main blood highway and into rest areas called adipose, or fat, cells. If the blockage continues, even more fat is stored in fat cells. This is something we want to avoid. Enter chromium. Chromium keeps the fat and sugar in our blood system pouring into muscle and brain cells where it gets burned off as energy—not stored as body fat.

Research Flash

The *Journal Of The American Medical Association* reports that chromium therapy was effective in fighting insulin resistance.

---

5. Corrects False Hunger Readings

Remember those really complicated Cold War spy stories, when each side released coded misinformation deliberately designed to confuse and cloud their real strategy. Something similar happens to our own internal fat communication system.

This is how it works. Our fat troubles don't just happen with too much insulin sending excessive blood fat into our fat cells. Our fat also accumulates when there is also too little insulin.

Insulin is responsible for sending the "I'm stuffed" message to our brain, shutting off the appetite control in our hypothalmus, located in our brain. If insulin levels are not kept on a fat regulating keel, your appetite control center never gets the "I'm stuffed" message.

Without chromium, misinformation is sent to our appetite control center—misinformation that says "more, more, more" when the real message should be "enough, enough, enough." Our appetite control center listens to the false message and we continue to stuff our faces with excess food—all of which gets stored as fat.

6. Boosts The Brown (Strawberry) Fat Burn

Remember strawberry fat? Chromium also stimulates our metabolic rate—the rate at which we burn calories for energy. As our metabolism speeds up, our body uses more energy. Because it uses more energy it sends out a call for more fuel. This is the process scientists call thermogenesis. And where does the "hottest" fat fuel come from? That's right. From our fat reserves. But not just any old fat reserves. Chromium helps reach way down into our strawberry fat reserves, tucked snug and deadly all along our our backs, and vital internal organs.

The Texas Study

In a double blind study a group taking chromium picolinate lost 4.2 pounds of fat and gained 1.4 pounds of muscle. The group not taking chromium picolinate had no fat loss or muscle gain.

When It's Not Fighting Fat, Chromium...

...**acts as a vascular scrubber,** lowering blood
triglycerides, (blood fat) lowering "bad"
LDL cholesterol, and raising "good" HDL.

...**helps reverse and prevent** Type II diabetes.

...**promotes** longevity.

...**impacts** on our immune system.

...**enhances** bio-energy.

...**improves** endurance.

....**increases** the level of DHEA in middle-aged
men and post-menopausal women.

...**builds** lean tissue of vital organs like the heart.

...**fights** fatigue.

...**stabilizes** mood swings.

...**protects** postmenopausal women from
osteoporosis and helps builds up estrogen.

The USDA Human Nutrition Research Center
found that chromium can lower blood sugar as
effectively as prescription medication,
without the side effects.

Older May Be Better
Studies show that people in their forties or fifties got better results from chromium picolinate supplemements than folks in their thirties.

Your Perfect Chromium Day

A combination of chromium from food sources and supplements is the scientific way to get maximum results.

Top Food Sources

Broccoli	Molasses
Brewer's yeast	Apples
Cereals	Beer
Grains	Prunes
Shellfish	Mushrooms
Liver	Wine
Kidneys	Eggs

Chromium No-No's

• High sugar content foods increase chromium excretion by up to 300%. Lose the chocolate, ketchup, sugary breakfast cereals, sodas.
• Food processing removes up to 80% of chromium.
• Physical stress.
• Air pollution.
• Change in hormone balance.
• Repeated pregnancies.

Supplements

The USDA admits that "there are no known foods eaten that are outstanding sources of dietary chromium." They report that sub-optimal chromium levels are common in the U.S. with ninety percent of Americans eating an average American diet receiving less than the RDA.

Dosage

National Research Council, National Academy of Science Recommendations.
Children

1 to 3 years old	20 to 80 mcg.
4 to 6 years old	30 to 120 mcg.
7 to 10 years old	50 to 100 mcg.
11+ years old	50 to 200 mcg.
Adults	50 to 200 mcg.

Possible Side Effects
Slight skin rash. Dizziness.

Best Form Of Chromium

Chromium picolinate is one of the forms that is best absorbed since it turns chromium into a form our bodies can use by helping the chromium slip through the cell membrane.

Chapter 6

Citrimax: The Fat Magician

Think about sucking on a freshly cut lemon, dripping and juicy. What happens? Your saliva gushes. Your taste-buds throb. Even your teeth pucker up. And that's just a plain old garden variety lemon.

Now think about a small, obscure fruit— round, wrinkled and sour enough to bring on an instant "pucker" hanging from a dusty tree in an ancient Calcutta orchard. Or piled high on a pungent dock in Thailand or in a noisy and steaming Burmese bazaar. Or peeled, sliced, and spread out in thin, translucent rows on a bamboo rack on the sandy shore of a Malaysian river.

That's garcinia cambogia, the strange and almost mystical fruit that has been eaten for centuries by over one half of the world and is now recognized as one of the most valuable treatments for contemporary obesity.

Thanks mainly to the efforts of ayurvedic physicians and healers who long recognized the value of garcinia cambogia, in the treatment of obesity, this wonderful fruit is now helping us shed our fat and find our natural and healthy appetite again.

Citrimax™ is the brand name for a highly effective formulation of garcinia cambogia.

Take the Garcinia Cambogia Challenge

1. I know I eat too much, but I can't seem to stop.
2. My cholesterol levels need to come down.
3. My appetite is out of control. I'm always hungry.

4. I'm uncomfortable with prescription drugs for appetite suppression and weight loss. I want something natural.
5. I don't want the risk of unpleasant side effects of prescription diet pills.
6. I want to lose more fat, faster.
7. I want to get a good night's sleep, without the tossing and wakefulness of many diet stimulants.
8. I want lots of energy.
9. I want to get rid of fatigue.
10. I want fat loss results that last.

Score: If you answered YES to even one of the above, you are a good candidate for one of nature's most gentle and effective fat loss nutrients.

Our Own Personal Rumplestiltskin Of Fat

Remember the story of the beautiful captive maiden locked in a musty dungeon by a greedy king who wouldn't let her out until she spun mountains of straw into gold for his treasury? But no matter how long she sat there, or how hard she wept, or how her fingers flew—straw in was still straw out. And then along comes Rumplestiltskin. This little gnome, who helps our heroine. And thanks to the magic powers of Rumplestiltskin—abracadabra—straw becomes gold!

Wouldn't it be nice if we had a personal Rumplestiltskin to turn our fat into lean? Or into energy? Into anything, but fat.

Now we have. It's called garcinia cambogia, or Citrimax™ nature's own fat magician.

The Four-In-One Fat Fighter

But seriously, there is no magic here. No story book Rumplestiltskin. Just great science. Great science that mounts a massive four pronged attack on our fat with just one little fruit.

1. Lipogenisis Inhibitor

Garcinia cambogia rinds contain hydroxycitric acid—HCA—a compound similar to the citric acid in our own familiar oranges, lemons and limes. So why not just go for what we know and grind up some grocery store citrus rind?

Because garcinia cambogia contains the most HCA. What's so special about HCA? Plenty.

Preliminary research indicates HCA decreases fat gain by inhibiting lipogenesis, the metabolic process by which our bodies turn food into fat. Here's how it works.

When you eat carbs they move into the digestive system where they are broken down into glucose—blood sugar—which our bodies use for energy. Any extra glucose that we don't need right away for digesting, breathing, thinking, driving, picking up the kids, watching TV, and occasionally jogging, gets stored in our liver and muscles. By the way, this extra glucose is now suddenly called glycogen—just like those annoying streets that seem to change their name every couple of miles through town until we are hopelessly lost.

When the liver and muscles get filled with glycogen, guess what? Another transformation. A pesky little enzyme, called citrate lyase or ATP rushes in and turns the glycogen into FAT!

That's where HCA steps in like a biological Mighty Mouse and blocks this enzyme fat maker from making fat. And fat is foiled again.

2. Lowers Blood Fat Levels

Researchers found that HCA lowers blood fat levels. This is also good. The less fat rushing through our vascular system, the less sticks to our arteries and the less messes with our insulin levels.

3. Appetite Control Central

Researchers found that HCA may help control appetite, resulting in fat loss without the loss of lean muscle tissue or body protein.

4. Thermogenesis Booster

Scientists believe that HCA may help stimulate fat loss by cranking up body heat production, (thermogenesis). Garcinia cambogia may jump start the process of burning up "hot" brown (strawberry) fat, which burns hotter and produces more body heat than garden variety yellow (vanilla) fat.

This brownish-pink fat is tucked around our vital organs to keep them warm—like that pink insulation we stuff into our attics. Its tint is caused by blood vessels and the energy rods called mitochondria that are our cellular fat furnaces. This type of fat is loaded with these powerful energy producers. Increasing the thermogenesis of brown (strawberry) fat helps overall weight loss.

What Makes Garcinia Cambogia A Great Fat Fighter?

First of all, garcinia cambogia is a real food, with very unique properties. It actually alters our fat and carbohydrate metabolism, without stimulating the central nervous system. The result? A more effective calorie burn without the "heebie jeebies" of other diet stimulants.

> Garcinia cambogia
> was a food for centuries before it became a modern fat fighter.
> It has a virtually unblemished safety record.

Recommended Daily Dose

300 mg taken daily with a full glass of water is the dose most often recommended.

Taking Garcinia cambogia with other fat fighters may enhance its fat fighting results.

Chapter 7

Chitosan: The Fat Sponge

Let's Make A Wish To The Fat Genie

Imagine. You have just scarfed down a double cheese burger, a large order of fries and a chocolate shake. Major guilt—not to mention—indigestion—sets in. You swear you can actually feel all that fat you just swallowed sticking to your hips, waist, belly and thighs.

You make a silent but desperate wish to the fat genie. "Please make some of this fat go away and I promise I'll never pig out again." Guess what? It's your lucky day. The fat genie has heard your wish and whispers back, "chitosan."

And chitosan it is. An almost magical supplement that can absorb four times its own weight in dietary fat, blocking it from entering your system. And if that weren't enough of a fat wish come true chitosan also attracts fat—binding with it in your tummy, before it passes through your digestive system and into your bloodstream--preventing it from being deposited on the insides of your arteries, around your heart and liver, and most especially around your waist, hips, arms, and thighs. That's some fat genie!

It All Started With A Mushroom

It all began a long time ago on a wonderful day in 1811 in France when Professor Henri Braconnot discovered a substance he called chitin—in a bunch of mushrooms.

Several years later, the same substance, chitin, was also isolated from insects. Later still, chitin was discovered in the shells of shrimp, lobsters, crabs and other shell fish.

What was this new substance called chitin? It turned out that chitin was a natural fiber. It was very similar to cellulose, found in many plants, and characterized by long graceful chains of molecules of N-acetyl-D-glucosamine.

It wasn't until over forty years later in 1859 in a different French laboratory, that another scientist, Professor C. Rouget, took an ordinary batch of chitin and "cooked" it in alkali. You would think that all he got was a mess of cooked chitin. Wrong. Here's where the true miracle of fat fighting science took place. The "cooked" chitin turned into one of nature's fiercest fat fighting warriors—chitosan.

"...Fire Burn And Cauldron Bubble"

What happened that day on that French professor's old stove? When the raw chitin was cooked it became deacetylated, which simply means that the acetyl parts of the chitin were pulled away leaving the glucosamine parts in their long wavy molecular chains. Chitin had become chitosan and chitosan would be found to have amazing fat fighting properties.

Chitosan As A Fat Magnet

Here's where the fat magnet part comes in. All molecules have either a positive or a negative charge. And if you remember anything at all from your high school science class you'll remember that opposites attract...for some of us that's true even when we aren't thinking about physics, right? Well, when the good professor pulled the chitosan chain out of the alkali "soup" he'd cooked it in, he found it had a positive charge. Stay with me. I'm almost done and think how you'll be able to impress your friends with all your newly acquired "fat physics." Guess what? Fat has a negative charge. The result? Chitosan and fat are attracted to each other. More than attracted. They stick together. Whenever chitosan comes anywhere near a fat molecule, it grabs on and doesn't let go. Like a magnet.

All kinds of fat stick to chitosan. Among the type of fat it attracts is the fat in bile acids containing cholesterol. When chitosan attracts bile acids, it increases the rate at which LDL is lowered and improves the ratio between LDL and HDL.

Chitosan packs a double fat fighting whammy. It's a **fat magnet**, attracting fat before it gets digested and a **fat sponge**, absorbing over 4 times its own weight in dietary fat.

Chitosan As Fat Blocker

Now, hooked up as it is with its new buddy, chitosan, your typical fat molecule, the one you just swallowed along with that burger, fries and shake, is way too big to pass through the delicate lining of your intestine. Too big to swim out of your tummy and into your bloodstream to clog up your veins and arteries with fatty sludge. Too big to pass through to wrap itself in thick layers around your heart and other vital organs. Too big to wad around your arms, thighs, waist, hips, chin.

Think Chitosan—Think Plastic Wrap For Fat

Chitosan has a netting effect, wrapping itself around fat droplets and preventing them from being digested by lipid enzymes. So what happens to this double-decker chitosan-fat combo? It becomes this nondigestible blob that passes through your system and right out of your body into the waste where it belongs. The result? Less fat sticks to you.

Chitosan is lipophilic which means it's a fat lover.

Fat Studies

There have been many chitosan studies including one of the first at Texas A & M University in 1983, another in Norway in 1991, in Japan in 1994 and this remarkable study:

The time. 1994.

The place. Finland.

The scientists. Professors Lasus and Abelin.

The question. Does chitosan work?

The results. WOW!

Thirty obese patients were given chitosan while a control group with an identical diet was given a placebo. In just four weeks the chitosan group lost an average of 15 pounds each compared to only 5 ½ pounds for the control group. The Finnish researchers reported that chitosan, "was the best and most hygenic way to take a weight-reducing substance."

Do The Fat Math
250 mg of chitosan absorbs 1000 mg of fat!

Take the Chitosan Challenge

1. I need something to jump start my diet.
2. I would like to lower my total cholesterol.
3. I want to reduce my risk for colon cancer.
4. I need to raise my HDL levels.
5. I suffer from indigestion, frequently.
6. I eat in fast food places several times a week.
7. I need to lose body fat.
8. I hate veggies.
9. I'm basically a meat & potatoes kind of person.
10. I've noticed I have more cavities than usual.

Score: If you answered YES to even one of these points you are a very good candidate for the fat fighter chitosan.

Chitosan At Work

Blocking fat and absorbing fat is just part of the miracle of chitosan. Studies show that this wonderful natural fiber has some remarkable additional properties...

...**protects** against the formation of many

cancers including breast, colon, rectum, pancreas and prostate cancer.

...**reduces** the risk of developing diabetes.

...**prevents** the formation of gall stones and kidney stones.

...**lowers** blood pressure.

...**alleviates** the risk and discomfort of arthritis.

...**soothes** ulcers.

...**speeds** the healing of wounds and broken bones.

...**slows** the formation of plaque that causes cavities.

Chitosan & Cholesterol

A study reported in the *American Journal of Clinical Nutrition* found that chitosan is as effective in mammals as cholestryramine—a cholesterol lowering drug—in controlling blood serum cholesterol without the negative side effects of the drug. Chitosan lowered blood cholesterol levels by 66.2 percent.

Chitosan reduces the levels of "bad cholesterol" or LDL and improves the ratio between LDL and "good cholesterol" or HDL.

Every time your total cholesterol level drops by 1% your risk of a heart attack drops by 2%. You do the math. Drop 5% and you lower your heart attack risk by an impressive 10%.

Chitosan Supplements

Daily 250 mg daily.
Take with 8 ounces of water.

Chitosan does not add any calories.

When Should I Take My Chitosan?

The best time to take your chitosan is between breakfast and lunch or before you know you are going to eat a high fat meal.

Warnings

Like any supplement you need to be careful about certain things. If you are allergic to shell fish, if you are pregnant or nursing, or if you are under the age of fourteen, DO NOT take chitosan. Because chitosan can bind with fat soluble vitamins such as vitamin E, A, D, and K, take those vitamins in the evening. In some people, chitosan may cause constipation or diarrhea.

Chitosan Boosters

Chitosan is pretty remarkable all by itself, but it's fat fighting power can be boosted with other nutrients.

Remember, chitosan is a fiber. And fibers can be sort of like a tangled chain which needs to be unravelled to work its fat fighting magic. The chitosan fiber chain has little fat hooks on each of the links that grab up fat molecules. In order to grab up as many fat molecules on the chitosan fat hooks it helps to make sure that the chain is stretched out to its full length without any tangles.

There are certain substances that help untangle the chitin chain and free up more fat hooks.

Vitamin C

When chitosan teams up with the powerhouse antioxidant vitamin C scientists report it may block a full 50 percent more fat.

Indoles

These are phytochemicals found in soy products. You may have heard of their ability to balance estrogen metabolism. But they also have the ability to prepare dietary toxins for elimination.

Garcinia Cambogia aka Citrimax™

Garcinia cambogia contains hydroxycitrate—HCA—a fat inhibitor with the ability to alter fat and carbohydrate metabolism and impact positively on weight loss.

Chapter 8

Citrus Aurantium: The Fat Fruit

A Mediterranean Miracle

Picture the scene. A warm sky above. The soft blue sea below. You sit in a tiny café overlooking a dusty square sipping espresso. A hard dry berry drops onto your table. Then another. And another. You ask their name. The waiter shrugs, "Bitter orange" and swipes them onto the patio tiles with a flick of his napkin. Little do you realize that those berries dropping from the slender, fragrant trees planted in thick terra cotta pots all around the café patio are one of the most powerful fat loss enhancers.

Those ancient trees, growing in Spain, Italy and Portugal and in parts of the West Indies, sprout berry-like fruit containing a substance called *zhi shi*. For thousands of years, Chinese healers extracted *zhi shi* from the immature dried fruit of the plant they called bitter orange and used the extracted powder to treat bouts of indigestion.

Centuries later, Western medicine would christen the plant, citrus aurantium and use its fruit to treat digestive and circulatory problems and as a natural and soothing sedative.

Neither East nor West realized the true power of that fragrant Mediterranean tree. Until now. Here is a powerful fat fighter.

Take The Citrus Aurantium Challenge

1. My metabolism seems to be slowing down and I want to give it a boost.
2. I want to get better results from my workouts.
3. I want to lose weight faster.
4. I want to take diet supplements that are completely natural.
5. I have high blood pressure.
6. My doctor told me to lose weight for my health.

7. Diets don't work for me.
8. I have trouble sleeping at night.
9. I eat on the run at least three times a week.
10.I seem to be stuck on a plateau and can't lose any more weight.

Scoring: If you answered YES to even one of these points, citrus aurantium may be just the right nutritional fat fighter to support your overall fat loss program.

Citrus Aurantium As Fat Buster

Like other fat fighting nutrients, citrus aurantium fights fat on more than one front and in more than one way.

Unlocks Fat Cells

Every single one of our body cells has an alphabet soup of receptors attached to its outside shell or membrane. Sort of like satellite dishes. Each one of these receptors is tuned into a different channel—programmed to receive a different message—a different set of instructions about what that cell should be doing next.

There's the twin receptors, Alpha-1 and Alpha-2 programmed to tighten and relax our veins and arteries. This duo is partly responsible for our blood pressure.

There's Beta-1 and Beta-2, two receptors which control cardiac function including heart rate.

Then, there's Beta-3, very important receptors—in the fat fight—and my personal favorites.

Beta-3 receptors are mostly clustered on the outside rim of fat cells and liver cells—both major fat storage tanks. Triggering Beta-3 receptors can make a significant difference in your ability to lose fat or not lose fat. Beta-3 receptors have three big jobs in our own cellular fat fight.

Fat Busting Job #1: Beta-3 speeds up the rate at which fat is released from body fat storage (a process called lipolysis).

Fat Busting Job #2: Beta-3 increases your resting metabolism, (a process called thermogenesis), accelerating the rate at which your body burns fat supplies even while you just sit around being a couch potato.

Fat Busting Job #3: Beta-3, through a series of chemical reactions, is able to stimulate the growth of muscle cells. And the more lean muscle tissue we have, the more energy we use and the more fat we burn.

Enter Citrus Aurantium

When a message is sent to our cells each one of these receptors picks it up—kind of like a huge community antenna. This is not always a good thing. Sometimes, we want to send a signal to only one of these receptors—Beta-3 for example—without turning on the others. All we want to do is dump fat and turn up our resting energy, right? And that's exactly what scientists believe citrus aurantium can do. They believe it zeros in on Beta-3 receptors only, turning on their powerful fat fighting signal, without stimulating the receptors that change heart rate or blood pressure. Preliminary research confirms, that unlike many other thermogenic products, citrus aurantium has no negative cardiovascular side effects—just positive fat fighting ones. The result? More fat is burned off as energy fuel. More energy means a higher bio-temperature and more calories burned even when we are completely at rest. More lean muscle is also retained and increased to keep that fat burn going strong.

Safety Issues

Citrus aurantium, scientists say, has no negative side effects. Its unique chemical composition makes it difficult for citrus aurantium molecules to cross the blood-brain barrier and so it cannot upset the delicate central nervous system, or the cardiovascular system.

Dosage

There is no RDA for citrus aurantium but a daily dose of 300 mg providing 4% synephrine is advised. Take it between breakfast and lunch with a full glass of water.

Part Three

The Skinny Food Clock

Chapter 9

Skinny Foods

For a long time many of us believed (based on our own experience) that pretty much all food is fat food. That there is no skinny food. Carrots or carrot cake it makes no difference, both turn into fat. Cottage cheese or cream pie, just fat waiting to happen. So why bother?

We usually begin to believe this somewhere between the salad and plain grilled hamburger patty we had for lunch (while trying to be good) and the cheese-topped baked potato and oatmeal-raisin cookies we had for dinner.

The irony is, if we just reversed the order of what we ate, we would find that indeed there is skinny food and we are already eating it! But we are eating it in the wrong order and at the wrong times of the day. And better yet, we aren't eating enough of it. That's right. If we just ate the cheese-topped baked potato and oatmeal raisin cookies for lunch, and had the plain grilled hamburger patty and salad for dinner—and another hamburger patty for a bedtime snack we would be well on our way to getting skinnier and healthier with every meal! And this is the revolutionary new principle behind the *Skinny Food Clock*. You don't believe me? Here, I'll show you.

Is There Anything I Can Eat That DOESN'T Turn Into Fat?

We have eaten cabbage soup and pineapples for weeks at a time. We have swallowed nasty shakes. Survived on macrobiotic brown rice. Switched to grapefruit. We have filled our lives with little plastic baggies bulging with veggie sticks, mixed nuts, mixed fruits and mixed cereal. We lost. We plateaued. We regained. We haven't enjoyed a meal since we were ten years old.

And now we scream in silence—is there anything out there we CAN eat? Anything that won't turn into fat? The answer is YES!

Skinny Foods That Fight Fat

A growing number of national and international sources—studies and research data—have begun to break the food-to-fat cycle in our daily diets. Here's what the newest research shows. There are two kinds of foods that fight fat.

There are Fat Blocker Foods.

There are Fat Burner Foods.

The Skinny Food Clock gives you plenty of both—seven times a day.

The Skinny Food Clock **Daily**

You will eat FAT BLOCKERS and FAT BURNERS in a very specific order.

When the clock says A.M. you will eat FAT BLOCKERS.

When the clock says P.M. you will eat FAT BURNERS.

That's it.
SIMPLE.
HEALTHY.
SKINNY!

Fat Blockers A.M.
Fat Burners P.M.

A.M. Foods = Fat Blocker Foods

Dietary fat blocking through food is a fascinating and tasty process that consists of two types of foods. *The Skinny Food Clock*, makes sure that you eat plenty of the Fat Blocking Foods and that you eat them when the clock says A.M. so that they can work to block any new dietary fat you may consume throughout the day.

Now, let's take a look at the two major categories of fat blocking skinny foods and how they work.

1. Foods that score high on the fullness index.
   These are foods that satisfy our hunger pangs without charging us a lot of fat-filling calories. These foods are high in fiber and carbs.

2. Foods that contain lots of fat-blocking fiber.
   Fiber is a key fat-blocking element that helps move dietary fat through our digestive system and transports it out, before it can be absorbed by our body and stored as fat.

The Fullness Index Foods

Our hunger is often the first thing that sabotages any fat reduction program. We've all been there. The growling tummy. The hollow, sinking feeling. The emptiness. The sudden fatigue. The inability to concentrate. The flash of irritability. All symptoms of hunger, whether real or imagined.

The response to these symptoms? Food. The faster the better.

But what food? How long will it soothe our hunger? How much will it cost us in empty calories?

Part of that answer comes from the Land Down Under—Australia. Researchers at the *University of Sydney* found that some foods make us feel fuller, more satisfied, and that the feeling of fullness lasted longer. What are these foods? And what part do they play in *The Skinny Food Clock* to block our own daily fat attacks?

The Australians were looking for the bargain foods, the foods that fill you up and keep you feeling fuller without having you pay a heavy price in calories.

Their findings are among the most exciting nutritional research in recent years. Here's what they did.

Australian researchers took a bunch of students and gave each of them a different food that contained 240 calories. Some kids got 240 calories worth of cake. Other kids got 240 calories worth of fish. Some got oatmeal or apples. Still others got 240 calories worth of croissants or potatoes or bananas.

Fifteen minutes after they ate their particular food they were asked to rate their feeling of fullness. Were they still full? Were they a little hungry? Were they famished? These ratings went on every fifteen minutes for the next two hours.

Then the real test began.

After two hours, all the students were set loose at a huge buffet table, and told to eat as much as they wanted.

Some of the students ate as if they hadn't seen food in years. Some ate a more-or-less average amount of food. And others just picked, saying they weren't really hungry.

What did the different students eat to give them such a varying appetite at the buffet table?

When the researchers finished compiling their data they made a very interesting discovery—interesting and crucial to our *Skinny Food Clock*.

Using white bread as ground zero, they found that certain foods do indeed have a higher satiety or fullness level than others.

The students who ate 240 calories worth of steak, for example, were not as hungry two hours later as the students who ate 240 calories worth of croissants.

So what are the fat fighting fullness foods and what role do they play in *The Skinny Food Clock*?

Here are the losers on the fullness index. These hardly fill you up at all. Whatever feelings of fullness you may have after eating them, don't last. And they are very expensive calorie-wise.

1. Croissant
2. Cake
3. Donut
4. Candy bar
5. Potato chips
6. Ice cream

The Fullness Index Winners

Here they are, foods that fill you up, keep you filled up and don't cost you too much in expensive calories ranked in order of their fullness index. Notice many of these foods are high in fiber and complex carbohydrates.

1. Potato
2. Oatmeal
3. Oranges
4. Apples
5. Pasta
6. Grapes
7. Popcorn
8. Bran cereal
9. Cheese
10. Crackers
11. Cookies
12. Bananas

Note: Steak and fish also scored high on the fullness index and are part of the P.M. fat burning foods in our *Skinny Food Clock* plan.

In *The Skinny Food Clock* these foods are arranged so that you eat lots of them in the early part of the day—when the clock says A.M. They fill you up fast. They keep you full. They don't use up precious calories. And they fight to stabilize and regulate your hunger and cravings so they don't sabotage your skinny progress.

Fiber Foods

Why do we hear and read so much about fat, protein and carbohydrates, but very little about fiber? What is fiber, anyway? And how does it fit into *The Skinny Food Clock* as a fat blocker?

Fiber Factoids

Fiber belongs to a branch of the carb family. Fiber is that part of complex carbohydrates that are not digested, but that pass right through our system and are excreted. Fiber has no calories. Great. It doesn't add to the dietary calories we can store as fat.

Fiber doesn't break down in our digestive system, which means it can't be absorbed, so again, it can't add to our fat supply. Fiber helps us feel full, soothing our appetite triggering center so that we are better able to refrain from stuffing ourselves. Fiber blocks the absorption of dietary fat –and fat calories—in our intestines and moves it harmlessly through our digestive system and out as waste. Fiber, as new research is showing every day, can help lower our blood fat, reducing cholesterol levels and improving our vascular health. It has also been shown to have a positive effect in reducing our risk for certain cancers and diabetes. Finally, most of us don't get nearly enough fiber every day—only 10 to 15 grams—as opposed to the 25 to 30 grams nutritional experts believe is the ideal and healthy amount.

Two Kinds Of Fat Blocking Fiber

There are two kinds of fat blocking fiber and we need both kinds.

Soluble Fiber: Think Gum

This is the fiber that dissolves in water, becoming sticky and gummy. It's the stickiness that attracts blood fat and cholesterol, pushing it out through your digestive system so it doesn't have a chance to be stored as fat. This is the fiber you think of when you think apples, oranges, broccoli, carrots, and potatoes. As it enters and passes through your system this soluble fiber helps lower cholesterol, reduces your risk for heart disease, improves blood sugar readings and in many cases helps lower blood pressure.

The Skinny Food Clock gives you lots of soluble fiber in your A.M. meals to help you fight fat all day long.

Insoluble Fiber: Think Sponge

This is the fiber you think of when you think of bran muffins, oat bran cereal, oatmeal or popcorn. When you eat this type of fiber and follow it with a big glass of water, the fiber swells up—like a sponge—absorbing the water. The now soft and spongy fiber pushes on and out through your intestines, carrying with it excess dietary fat. As it passes through you, studies show that it helps in your overall digestion, aids elimination, promotes regularity and helps keep bowels clean

The Skinny Food Clock gives you lots of insoluble fiber in your A.M. meals to help you fight fat all day long.

List Of A.M. Fat Blocker Foods

Apple
Apricot
Artichokes
Asparagus
Avocado
Banana
Beans (kidney)
Beans (lima)
Beets
Bread (pumpernickel)
Bread (seven-grain)
Broccoli
Buckwheat
Carrots
Chickpeas
Corn on the cob
Cucumber
Dates
Figs

Grapefruit
Green Beans
Lentils
Lettuce
Mushrooms
Oatmeal
Oat bran
Oranges
Pears
Pineapple
Popcorn
Potatoes
Prunes
Raisins
Raspberries
Rice
Spinach
Yams

P.M. Foods = Fat Burner Foods

We really can burn off stored calories—fat—while we eat! I know it sounds like one of those headlines you might read while waiting in your supermarket check-out line, but there really are foods that help burn fat.

Let's back up just a minute and look at the different ways our body burns off fat calories.

Our body burns fat calories off through our metabolic rate. Remember? That's the amount of calories our body needs every day, awake or asleep to run our basic metabolic functions. We already know that one way to increase our metabolic rate and burn more fat for energy is to increase our physical activity. Simple.

Now here's another way. We can increase our metabolic rate through a diet high in thermic foods. Yes, we can actually burn more calories WHILE WE EAT! Look at it this way. Our own body is our best fat burning machine. Just at rest, doing nothing more strenuous than keeping us breathing and blinking our body uses up to 60 percent of the calories we consume.

Any amount of physical exercise we do uses up another 25 percent of our calories. That leaves 15 percent. And that's a critical part of *The Skinny Food Clock.*

Activity	% of Calories Burned Off
Resting metabolic rate	60%
Physical exercise	25%
THERMIC FOODS	15%

Here's the good news. The skinny news. By eating thermic foods—foods that produce heat—hot calorie foods—you can burn off 15 percent of your daily calories just in the caloric energy you use to eat, digest and most importantly, process thermic foods. Your metabolic rate increases when you eat these foods because your body has to work very hard to break down and absorb the nutrients in these foods. This produces more heat. More calories are burned off. Fewer calories are available to be stored as fat. This process is called the thermic effect of food. But not all foods produce the same thermic burn. Not all foods have fat burning hot calories

Hot Calorie Foods

Surprise. Surprise.

Fat has no hot calories. Fat is not a thermic food. When you eat 200 calories worth of dietary fat, or food fat, your body only uses up a pathetic 6 calories—or 3 percent—to process that fat. That leaves 194 calories that can go right into your fat storage.

Carbs are hot calorie foods. You burn more calories eating carbs than you burn eating fat. When you eat 200 carb calories, you burn off 46 calories just to process the nutrients. That's 23 percent.

Protein gives us the biggest thermic fat burn of all—using up more hot calories than fat or carbs. But until now, most of the protein we ate to get our fat burn came from red meat heavily laced with fat. The result? We weren't getting the maximum burn from the hot calorie protein.

With *The Skinny Food Clock*, your P.M. meals will be high protein—hot calorie—major fat burners, but without the heavy lacing of fat that undermines the burn.

List of P.M. Fat Burner Foods

Lean red meat
Chicken without skin
Turkey without skin
Lamb, trimmed
Pork, trimmed
Yogurt, nonfat, any flavor
Skim milk
Nonfat and/or lowfat cheese
Egg whites or egg substitutes
Tofu
Vegetarian meat substitutes

Part Four

Putting It All Together & Getting Skinny

Chapter 10

Putting It All Together

The 24 Hours That Will Start To Change Your Body Chemistry From Fat To Skinny

The Skinny Pill.

This fat fighting formula is a carefully designed supplement cocktail of the five key dietary supplements, carnitine, chromium, chitosan, citrimax and citrus aurantium, to fight your fat on a cellular or biochemical level.

You do not need a prescription for any of these fat fighting nutrients.

The five key fat fighters in *The Skinny Pill* will help your body block dietary fat, will work with your metabolism to boost the rate at which your body burns off fat stores, will lower your cravings and hunger pangs, will energize you and help reduce those dieting blues.

The Skinny Pill
Carnitine
Chromium
Citrimax
Chitosan
Citrus Aurantium

The Supporting Skinny Supplements

Unlike most plans *The Skinny Pill* and *The Skinny Food Clock* believe you need to supplement your daily food intake with nutritional supplements. But what to take? When to take them? How many? These are all questions we keep asking as we stuff little plastic baggies with our vitamins and minerals. No more. Your basic supporting nutritional supplements are included every single day. You will know exactly how to take them. What to take. And when.

Skinny Supporting Supplements
Calcium
Multivitamin and/or antioxidant blend

The Skinny Food Clock

7 Meals-A-Day

Each of the seven daily meals is carefully calculated and pre-designed to meet your daily nutritional and calorie requirements.

Your A.M. Fat Blockers

You will enjoy a pre-breakfast, a hearty breakfast, a morning snack and a generous lunch with an emphasis on fat blocking foods high in fiber. These A.M. foods will help your body block dietary fat.

Your P.M. Fat Burners

You will enjoy an afternoon snack, a wonderful dinner and an exciting bedtime snack with an emphasis on fat burning foods, high in protein. These P.M. foods will help your body burn off stored fat...even while you sleep.

Special Skinny Recipes

Did you ever think you would be eating a banana split for breakfast, oatmeal cookies for a snack, grilled steak for dinner and a generous deli platter of cold cuts at bedtime and still lose fat?
You will enjoy special recipes for breakfast, snacks, lunches, and dinner. In fact these skinny foods are so fantastic you will serve them to your whole family and to guests. And no-one will suspect that they will be burning unwanted fat with every delicious bite.

These specially developed skinny foods are integral to *The Skinny Pill* and *The Skinny Food Clock.*

Skinny Banana Split

1 banana, peeled and split lengthwise
1 orange, peeled and chopped
1 kiwi fruit, peeled and chopped
½ cup raspberries or strawberries.
1 big scoop nonfat frozen yogurt

Arrange the banana on a small plate or dish. Top with the frozen yogurt. Place the mixed fruit on the yogurt. Dig in and enjoy. Makes one serving.

Skinny Sundae

1 cup frozen nonfat yogurt
¼ cup bran cereal
½ cup raspberries or strawberries.
1 tablespoon chocolate syrup (optional)

In a tall parfait glass layer the fruit, yogurt and cereal in alternating layers. Top with the chocolate syrup. Enjoy. Makes one serving.

Skinny Cookies

½ cup oatmeal
½ cup oat bran
½ cup raisins
1 cup lowfat pancake mix
½ cup brown sugar
½ cup unsweetened applesauce
½ teaspoon cinnamon
4 to 6 packets artificial sweetener
½ cup water or enough to form cookie consistency

Preheat oven to 350°

Combine all ingredients in a medium bowl. Stir with a fork until well mixed. Drop by teaspoonfuls on a nonstick cookie sheet. Flatten slightly with the tines of a fork. Bake for 15 minutes or until golden brown. Let cool. Store in an airtight container in the fridge. Makes 1 dozen.
Two cookies = one serving.

Skinny Munchies

3 cups Total® cereal
3 cups hot-air popped popcorn
1 cup broken up whole wheat crackers
1 cup lightly salted pretzel sticks
2 tablespoons vegetable oil
½ teaspoon chili powder
¼ teaspoon ground cumin
1 teaspoon garlic powder
2 tablespoons grated Parmesan cheese

Preheat oven to 300°

Mix cereal, popcorn, crackers and pretzels in a large plastic bag. In a small bowl combine the oil and the spices. Pour over the dry mixture. Shake well. Immediately sprinkle with cheese. Shake well again. Pour into ungreased rectangular baking pan, 13 x 9 x 2-inches. Bake 10 minutes without stirring. Cool. Store in a tightly covered container. Makes 8 cups. 1 cup = 1 serving.

Skinny Salad

1 head Romaine lettuce, cleaned and chopped
1 bunch fresh spinach leaves, cleaned and chopped
2 bunches of scallions, chopped
4 stalks celery, chopped
1 red pepper, seeded and chopped
1 green pepper, seeded and chopped
1 tomato, chopped
1 bunch parsley, chopped

Combine all ingredients in a large plastic container. Store in fridge. 4 cups = 1 serving.

Skinny Fruit Salad

1 apple, cored but not peeled, chopped
1 pear, cored but not peeled, chopped
1 orange, peeled and seeded, chopped
1 cup raspberries, washed
1 cup blueberries, washed
1 pint strawberries, washed and hulled

Combine all fruit in a large bowl. Chill.
1 cup = 1 serving

Skinny Mixed Veggies

1 bag frozen peas
1 bag frozen carrots
1 bag frozen mini onions
1 bag frozen corn kernels

Keeping the veggies frozen, combine the peas, carrots and onions into one large freezer bag. Keep frozen until needed. 1 cup = 1 serving.

Skinny Steamed Veggies

1 large head broccoli, cut into flowerets
1 cauliflower, cut into flowerets
1 bag mini carrots

In a large plastic bag combine the veggies. Seal and keep in the fridge until used.
3 cups = 1 serving.

Skinny Deli Platter

3 slices nonfat ham or
3 slices nonfat turkey or
3 slices nonfat chicken
1 ounce nonfat cheese or
1 hard-boiled egg—white only
1 sliced tomato
2 large leaves Romaine lettuce

Arrange the meats and the egg and sliced tomato on the lettuce leaves. Enjoy! Makes one serving

Skinny Omelet

1 whole egg
2 egg whites
1 chopped scallion or ¼ cup chopped onion
3 slices nonfat ham, chopped fine
salt and pepper to taste
vegetable spray

Whisk the egg and egg white together in a bowl. Heat a nonstick omelet pan sprayed with vegetable spray. Lightly cook the chopped onion until soft and the ham until warm. Remove and keep warm. Add the egg to the pan. Cook until the bottom is set. Tilt the pan slightly until all the liquid egg runs under and sets. Sprinkle the ham and chopped onion on top and fold the egg over. Transfer to a plate. Garnish if you like with some sliced tomato or parsley or lettuce.
Makes one serving.

Skinny Servings Quick Reference Guide

Food	Serving Size
Skinny Banana Split	1 split
Skinny Sundae	1 sundae
Skinny Cookies	2 cookies
Skinny Munchies	1 cup
Skinny Salad	4 cups
Skinny Fruit Salad	1 cup
Skinny Mixed Veggies	1 cup
Skinny Steamed Veggies	3 cups
Skinny Deli Platter	1 platter
Skinny Omelet	1 omelet

Day 1

Pre-Breakfast
Apple or Pear or Orange. Pick one only

Breakfast
1 cup oatmeal with 2 teaspoons brown sugar
500 mg calcium

Morning Snack
1 cup nonfat fruit yogurt or frozen yogurt & ½ cantaloupe.
The Skinny Pill Formula with 12 ounces of water

Lunch
Individual can water-packed tuna and *Skinny Salad*

Afternoon Snack
3 ounces of nonfat cheese &1 serving jello with nonfat
whipped topping.

Dinner
Skinny Salad, Skinny Steamed Veggies, 8 oz lean steak
Multivitamin and/or antioxidant

Bedtime Snack
Skinny Omelet
500 mg calcium

Day 2

Pre-Breakfast
Apple or Pear or Orange. Pick one only.

Breakfast
½ bagel with 1 teaspoon all-fruit preserves or honey
500 mg calcium

Morning Snack
Skinny Cookies
The Skinny Pill Formula with 12 ounces water.

Lunch
½ bagel with 1 tsp. cream cheese and *Skinny Salad*

Afternoon Snack
Skinny Fruit Salad

Dinner
Skinny Salad, Skinny Steamed Veggies and 8 oz. fish,
baked or broiled
Multivitamin and/or antioxidant

Bedtime Snack
Skinny Omelet
500 mg calcium

Day 3

Pre-Breakfast
Apple or Pear or Orange. Pick one only.

Breakfast
1 cup Total® cereal & ½ cup skim milk & ¼ cup raisins
500 mg calcium

Morning Snack
Skinny Fruit Salad
The Skinny Pill Formula with 12 ounces of water

Lunch
1 hamburger patty, grilled with *Skinny Salad*

Afternoon Snack
2 stalks of celery with 1 tablespoon peanut butter

Dinner
Skinny Salad, Skinny Steamed Veggies and 8 oz. chicken
or turkey, skinless.
Multivitamin and/or antioxidant

Bedtime Snack
Skinny Deli Platter
500 mg calcium

Day 4

Pre-Breakfast
Apple or Pear or Orange. Pick one only.

Breakfast
2 slices toast with 2 tsp. all-fruit preserve
500 mg calcium

Morning Snack
1 cup nonfat fruit yogurt or 1 cup nonfat frozen yogurt
The Skinny Pill Formula with 12 ounces water

Lunch
Skinny Omelet with *Skinny Salad*

Afternoon Snack
3 oz. nonfat cheese & 1 cup assorted raw veggies

Dinner
Skinny Salad, Skinny Steamed Veggies and 8 oz. fish,
baked or broiled
Multivitamin and/or antioxidant

Bedtime Snack
Skinny Deli Platter
500 mg calcium

Day 5

Pre-Breakfast
Apple or Pear or Orange. Pick one only.

Breakfast
2 waffles with 2 teaspoons syrup or honey
500 mg calcium

Morning Snack
Skinny Fruit Salad
The Skinny Pill Formula with 12 ounces water

Lunch
Skinny Deli Platter with *Skinny Salad*

Afternoon Snack
3 ounces of nonfat cheese

Dinner
Skinny Salad, Skinny Steamed Veggies and 8 oz. lean
steak, baked or broiled
Multivitamin and/or antioxidant

Bedtime Snack
Skinny Omelet
500 mg calcium

Day 6

Pre-Breakfast
apple, orange, pear, or cup of raspberries. Pick one only.

Breakfast
1 cup oatmeal with 2 teaspoons brown sugar.
500 mg calcium.

Morning Snack
Skinny Cookies.
The Skinny Pill Formula with 12 ounces water

Lunch
1 cup pea or tomato soup.
1 pita bread stuffed with *Skinny Salad.*

Afternoon Snack
4 stalks celery with 1 tablespoon peanut butter.

Dinner
Skinny Salad. Skinny Veggie Mix. 8 ounces fish.
Multivitamin and/or antioxidant.

Bedtime Snack
Skinny Deli Platter.
500 mg calcium.

Day 7

Pre-Breakfast
apple, orange, pear, cup of raspberries. Pick one only.

Breakfast
Skinny Banana Split.
500 mg calcium.

Morning Snack
Skinny Munchies.
The Skinny Pill Formula with 12 ounces water

Lunch
1 cup vegetable soup with ½ bagel, *Skinny Salad.*

Afternoon Snack
½ cantaloupe.

Dinner
Skinny Salad. 8 ounces chicken breast. *Skinny Steamed Veggies.*
Multivitamin and/or antioxidant.

Bedtime Snack
Skinny Omelet.
500 mg calcium.

Day 8

Pre-Breakfast
apple, orange, pear, or cup of raspberries. Pick one only.

Breakfast
2 waffles with 2 teaspoons syrup.
500 mg calcium.

Morning Snack
Skinny Fruit Salad.
The Skinny Pill Formula with 12 ounces water.

Lunch
1 cup lentil soup. *Skinny Salad.*

Afternoon Snack
1 cup nonfat fruit yogurt or 1 cup nonfat frozen yogurt.

Dinner
Skinny Salad. 8 ounces steak. *Skinny Steamed Veggies.*
Multivitamin and/or antioxidant.

Bedtime Snack
3 ounces nonfat cheese. 1 cup sugar free jello with nonfat
dairy topping.
500 mg calcium.

Day 9

Pre-Breakfast

apple, orange, pear, or cup of raspberries. Pick one only.

Breakfast

Skinny Sundae.
500 mg calcium.

Morning Snack

Skinny Cookies.
The Skinny Pill Formula with 12 ounces water.

Lunch

1 cup pasta with marinara or primavera sauce.
Skinny Salad.

Afternoon Snack

Skinny Fruit Salad.

Dinner

Skinny Salad. Skinny Mixed Veggies. Skinny Omelet.
Multivitamin and/or antioxidant.

Bedtime Snack

Skinny Deli Platter.
500 mg calcium.

Day 10

Pre-Breakfast
apple, orange, pear, or cup of raspberries. Pick one only.

Breakfast
1 cup whole grain cereal with ½ cup skim milk.
500 mg calcium.

Morning Snack
Skinny Munchies.
The Skinny Pill Formula with 12 ounces water.

Lunch
1 glass tomato juice. 1 cup vegetable chili. 1 pita bread.

Afternoon Snack
½ cantaloupe.

Dinner
Skinny Salad. 8 ounces broiled steak.
Skinny Steamed Veggies.
Multivitamin and/or antioxidant.

Bedtime Snack
1 individual can water-packed tuna. *Skinny Salad.*
500 mg calcium.

Day 11

Pre-Breakfast

apple, orange, pear, or cup of raspberries. Pick one only.

Breakfast

Skinny Banana Split.
500 mg calcium.

Morning Snack

Skinny Cookies.
The Skinny Pill Formula with 12 ounces water.

Lunch

1 cup bean with bacon soup. *Skinny Salad.*

Afternoon Snack

1 cup jello with nonfat whipped topping.
1 ounce lowfat or nonfat cheese.

Dinner

Skinny Salad. 8 ounces turkey breast.
Sliced tomato and onion.
Multivitamin and/or antioxidant.

Bedtime Snack

Skinny Omelet.
500 mg calcium.

Day 12

Pre-Breakfast

apple, orange, pear, or cup of raspberries. Pick one only.

Breakfast

2 pancakes with 2 teaspoons syrup.
500 mg calcium.

Morning Snack

3 cups air-popped popcorn.
The Skinny Pill Formula with 12 ounces water.

Lunch

Skinny Omelet. 1 glass vegetable juice.

Afternoon Snack

½ cantaloupe.

Dinner

Skinny Mixed Veggies. 8 ounces fish.
1 cup coleslaw with nonfat dressing.
Multivitamin and/or antioxidant.

Bedtime Snack

Skinny Deli Platter
500 mg calcium.

Day 13

Pre-Breakfast
apple, orange, pear, or cup of raspberries. Pick one only.

Breakfast
1 cup oatmeal with 2 teaspoons brown sugar.
500 mg calcium.

Morning Snack
Skinny Cookies.
The Skinny Pill Formula with 12 ounces water.

Lunch
1 cup pea or lentil soup. *Skinny Salad.*

Afternoon Snack
4 stalks celery with 1 tablespoon peanut butter.

Dinner
Skinny Salad. Skinny Veggie Mix. 8 ounces fish.
Multivitamin and/or antioxidant.

Bedtime Snack
Skinny Deli Platter.
500 mg calcium.

Day 14

Pre-Breakfast

apple, orange, pear, cup of raspberries. Pick one only.

Breakfast

Skinny Banana Split.
500 mg calcium.

Morning Snack

Skinny Munchies.
The Skinny Pill Formula with 12 ounces water.

Lunch

1 cup tomato soup with ½ bagel and *Skinny Salad.*

Afternoon Snack

½ cantaloupe.

Dinner

Skinny Salad. 8 ounces chicken breast.
Skinny Steamed Veggies.
Multivitamin and/or antioxidant. 8 oz water.

Bedtime Snack

Skinny Omelet.
500 mg calcium.

Day 15

Pre-Breakfast
apple, orange, pear, or cup of raspberries. Pick one only.

Breakfast
2 waffles with 2 teaspoons syrup.
500 mg calcium. 8 oz water.

Morning Snack
Skinny Fruit Salad.
The Skinny Pill Formula with 12 ounces water.

Lunch
1 cup lentil soup. *Skinny Salad.*

Afternoon Snack
1 cup nonfat fruit yogurt or 1 cup nonfat frozen yogurt.

Dinner
Skinny Salad. 8 ounces steak. *Skinny Steamed Veggies.*
Multivitamin and/or antioxidant.

Bedtime Snack
3 ounces nonfat cheese. 1 cup sugar free jello with nonfat
dairy topping.
500 mg calcium.

Day 16

Pre-Breakfast
apple, orange, pear, or cup of raspberries. Pick one only.

Breakfast
2 slices bread toasted with 2 teaspoons all fruit preserves.
500 mg calcium. 8 oz water.

Morning Snack
Skinny Cookies.
The Skinny Pill Formula with 12 ounces water.

Lunch
1 cup pasta with marinara or primavera sauce.
Skinny Salad.

Afternoon Snack
½ cantaloupe

Dinner
Skinny Salad. Skinny Mixed Veggies. Skinny Omelet.
Multivitamin and/or antioxidant.

Bedtime Snack
Skinny Deli Platter.
500 mg calcium.

Day 17

Pre-Breakfast
apple, orange, pear, or cup of raspberries. Pick one only.

Breakfast
1 cup whole grain cereal with ½ cup skim milk.
500 mg calcium.

Morning Snack
Skinny Munchies.
The Skinny Pill Formula with 12 ounces water.

Lunch
1 glass tomato juice. 1 cup vegetable chili.

Afternoon Snack
½ cantaloupe.

Dinner
Skinny Salad. 8 ounces broiled steak.
Skinny Steamed Veggies.
Multivitamin and/or antioxidant.

Bedtime Snack
1 individual can water-packed tuna. *Skinny Salad.*
500 mg calcium.

Day 18

Pre-Breakfast

apple, orange, pear, or cup of raspberries. Pick only one.

Breakfast

Skinny Banana Split.
500 mg calcium.

Morning Snack

Skinny Cookies.
The Skinny Pill Formula with 12 ounces water.

Lunch

1 cup bean with bacon soup. 1 pita bread with *Skinny Salad.*

Afternoon Snack

1 cup sugar free jello with nonfat dairy topping.

Dinner

Skinny Salad. 8 ounces roast turkey breast.
Sliced tomato and onion.
Multivitamin and/or antioxidant.

Bedtime Snack

Skinny Omelet.
500 mg calcium.

Day 19

Pre-Breakfast

apple, orange, pear, or cup of raspberries. Pick only one.

Breakfast

2 pancakes with 2 teaspoons syrup.
500 mg calcium.

Morning Snack

3 cups air-popped popcorn.
The Skinny Pill Formula with 12 ounces water.

Lunch

1 can individual tuna with nonfat dressing. 1 glass
vegetable juice.

Afternoon Snack

3 ounces nonfat cheese.

Dinner

Skinny Mixed Veggies. 8 ounces fish.
1 cup coleslaw with nonfat dressing.
Multivitamin and/or antioxidant.

Bedtime Snack

Skinny Deli Platter
500 mg calcium.

Day 20

Pre-Breakfast

apple, orange, pear, or cup of raspberries. Pick only one.

Breakfast

Skinny Omelet.
500 mg calcium.

Morning Snack

3 ounces nonfat cheese.
The Skinny Pill Formula with 12 ounces water.

Lunch

Skinny Salad.
1 cup nonfat fruit yogurt or 1 cup nonfat frozen yogurt.

Afternoon Snack

4 stalks celery with 1 tablespoon peanut butter.

Dinner

Skinny Salad. Skinny Steamed Veggies.. 8 ounces fish.
Multivitamin and/or antioxidant.

Bedtime Snack

Skinny Deli Platter.
500 mg calcium.

Day 21

Pre-Breakfast
Apple or Pear or Orange. Pick one only.

Breakfast
2 waffles with 2 teaspoons syrup or honey
500 mg calcium

Morning Snack
Skinny Fruit Salad
The Skinny Pill Formula with 12 ounces water

Lunch
Skinny Deli Platter with *Skinny Salad*

Afternoon Snack
3 ounces of nonfat cheese

Dinner
Skinny Salad, Skinny Steamed Veggies and 8 oz. lean
steak, baked or broiled
Multivitamin and/or antioxidant

Bedtime Snack
Skinny Omelet
500 mg calcium

Day 22

Pre-Breakfast
apple, orange, pear, or cup of raspberries. Pick one only.

Breakfast
1 cup oatmeal with 2 teaspoons brown sugar.
500 mg calcium.

Morning Snack
Skinny Cookies.
The Skinny Pill Formula with 12 ounces water

Lunch
1 cup pea or tomato soup. *Skinny Salad.*

Afternoon Snack
4 stalks celery with 1 tablespoon peanut butter.

Dinner
Skinny Salad. Skinny Veggie Mix. 8 ounces fish.
Multivitamin and/or antioxidant.

Bedtime Snack
Skinny Deli Platter.
500 mg calcium.

Day 23

Pre-Breakfast

apple, orange, pear, cup of raspberries. Pick one only.

Breakfast

Skinny Banana Split.
500 mg calcium.

Morning Snack

Skinny Munchies.
The Skinny Pill Formula with 12 ounces water

Lunch

1 cup vegetable soup. *Skinny Salad.*

Afternoon Snack

½ cantaloupe.

Dinner

Skinny Salad. 4 ounces chicken breast. *Skinny Steamed Veggies.*
Multivitamin and/or antioxidant. 8 oz water.

Bedtime Snack

Skinny Omelet.
500 mg calcium.

Day 24

Pre-Breakfast
apple, orange, pear, or cup of raspberries. Pick one only.

Breakfast
2 waffles with 2 teaspoons syrup.
500 mg calcium.

Morning Snack
Skinny Fruit Salad.
The Skinny Pill Formula with 12 ounces water.

Lunch
1 cup lentil soup. *Skinny Salad.*

Afternoon Snack
1 cup nonfat fruit yogurt or 1 cup nonfat frozen yogurt.

Dinner
Skinny Salad. 8 ounces steak. *Skinny Steamed Veggies.*
Multivitamin and/or antioxidant.

Bedtime Snack
3 ounces nonfat cheese. *Skinny Salad.*
500 mg calcium.

Day 25

Pre-Breakfast

apple, orange, pear, or cup of raspberries. Pick one only.

Breakfast

2 slices bread toasted with 2 teaspoons all fruit preserves.
500 mg calcium.

Morning Snack

Skinny Cookies.
The Skinny Pill Formula with 12 ounces water.

Lunch

1 cup pasta with marinara or primavera sauce.
Skinny Salad.

Afternoon Snack

½ cantaloupe.

Dinner

Skinny Salad. Skinny Mixed Veggies. Skinny Omelet.
Multivitamin and/or antioxidant.

Bedtime Snack

Skinny Deli Platter.
500 mg calcium.

Day 26

Pre-Breakfast

apple, orange, pear, or cup of raspberries. Pick one only.

Breakfast

1 cup whole grain cereal with ½ cup skim milk.
500 mg calcium.

Morning Snack

Skinny Munchies.
The Skinny Pill Formula with 12 ounces water.

Lunch

1 glass tomato juice. 1 cup vegetable chili. 1 pita bread.

Afternoon Snack

½ cantaloupe.

Dinner

Skinny Salad. 8 ounces broiled steak.
Skinny Steamed Veggies.
Multivitamin and/or antioxidant.

Bedtime Snack

1 individual can water-packed tuna. 3 ounces nonfat
cheese.
500 mg calcium.

Day 27

Pre-Breakfast

apple, orange, pear, or cup of raspberries. Pick one only.

Breakfast

Skinny Banana Split.
500 mg calcium.

Morning Snack

Skinny Cookies.
The Skinny Pill Formula with 12 ounces water.

Lunch

1 cup bean with bacon soup. 1 pita bread with *Skinny Salad.*

Afternoon Snack

1 ounce lowfat or nonfat cheese. 1 cup sugar free jello with nonfat whipped topping.

Dinner

Skinny Salad. 8 ounces roast turkey breast.
Sliced tomato and onion.
Multivitamin and/or antioxidant.

Bedtime Snack

Skinny Omelet.
500 mg calcium.

Day 28

Pre-Breakfast

apple, orange, pear, or cup of raspberries. Pick one only.

Breakfast

2 pancakes with 2 teaspoons syrup.
500 mg calcium.

Morning Snack

3 cups air-popped popcorn.
The Skinny Pill Formula with 12 ounces water.

Lunch

Skinny Deli Platter. 1 glass vegetable juice.

Afternoon Snack

1 cup strawberries with nonfat whipped topping.

Dinner

Skinny Mixed Veggies. 8 ounces fish.
1 cup coleslaw with nonfat dressing.
Multivitamin and/or antioxidant.

Bedtime Snack

Skinny Deli Platter
500 mg calcium.

Day 29

Pre-Breakfast
apple, orange, pear, or cup of raspberries. Pick one only.

Breakfast
1 cup oatmeal with 2 teaspoons brown sugar.
500 mg calcium.

Morning Snack
Skinny Cookies.
The Skinny Pill Formula with 12 ounces water.

Lunch
1 cup pea or lentil soup. 1 pita bread with *Skinny Salad.*

Afternoon Snack
4 stalks celery with 1 tablespoon peanut butter.

Dinner
Skinny Salad. Skinny Veggie Mix. 8 ounces fish.
Multivitamin and/or antioxidant.

Bedtime Snack
Skinny Deli Platter.
500 mg calcium.

Day 30

Pre-Breakfast
apple, orange, pear, cup of raspberries. Pick one only.

Breakfast
Skinny Banana Split.
500 mg calcium.

Morning Snack
Skinny Munchies.
The Skinny Pill Formula with 12 ounces water.

Lunch
1 cup tomato soup with ½ bagel and *Skinny Salad.*

Afternoon Snack
½ cantaloupe.

Dinner
Skinny Salad. 8 ounces chicken breast.
Skinny Steamed Veggies.
Multivitamin and/or antioxidant. 8 oz water.

Bedtime Snack
Skinny Omelet.
500 mg calcium.

Part Five

Keeping The Skinny Going

Chapter 11

Staying Skinny

The M Word. Maintenance. You've done it. You are finally winning your personal war on fat. Your clothes fit better—you're even interested in shopping again. Your old scale confirms the steady downward slide—recording lost fat pounds quickly and permanently. You have good muscle tone. You have definition. You have more energy. You feel better. You are moving out of the high risk category for heart disease, stroke, cancers and diabetes. If you go to your doctor for a check-up now, there is a good chance that your cholesterol levels will have dropped, that your ratio of "good" cholesterol (HDL) to "bad" cholesterol (LDL) will have improved and that your blood pressure will be in a healthier range.

Now, the idea is to keep winning the fat fight. You've got the basics. You've got the idea. You have seen what works and how. You can do it. You can keep it going.

Just remember the basics.

1. *The Skinny Pill*
2. *The Skinny Food Clock*
   A.M. Foods To Block Fat
   P.M. Foods To Burn Fat

Making Your Own Skinny Selections

While I prefer that you follow the daily menus exactly as I have laid out until you get very comfortable and really understand how the A.M. fat blocking and P.M. fat burning foods work, I do understand that sometimes you may have a preference for a certain food, an intense dislike of another food, or you may just be in a position where you can't stick to my selections exactly. If this should happen, please feel free to make your selections from the categories and choices below. And don't worry. Even if you make a few personal choices to replace the ones I'm suggesting, you will not jeopardize your own journey to Skinny.

Pre-Breakfast

Chose only ONE

Apple
Pear
Orange
1 cup raspberries
No other choices are permitted

Breakfast

Choose only ONE

Skinny Banana Split
Skinny Sundae
2 waffles
2 pancakes
½ bagel, any kind
2 slices toast, any kind of bread
1 cup oatmeal, prepared in water
1 serving whole bran cereal, such as Total®
1 cup oat bran cereal
1 cup cream of wheat cereal
1 cup cooked grits (no butter or cheese please)

You may also have one of the following at breakfast: 2 teaspoons all-fruit preserves, jam, jelly, 2 teaspoons cream cheese, syrup, brown sugar, white sugar, honey or artificial sweetener.
½ cup skim milk, low fat soy or rice beverage.

(Hint try using 1 teaspoon of cream cheese and 1 teaspoon of all-fruit preserves on your bread or ½ bagel)

Morning Snack

Chose only ONE

Skinny cookies
Skinny munchies
Skinny fruit salad
3-cups air-popped popcorn
1 cup pretzels
¼ cup raisins
¼ cup dried apple slices
6 small graham crackers
8 animal crackers
2 fig cookies
1 apple
1 pear
1 orange
1 cup raspberries
1 cup blueberries
1 cup strawberries
½ cantaloupe
½ cup rice pudding made with skim milk
½ cup pudding made with skim milk
1 cup jello with nonfat whipped topping
1 cup frozen yogurt or lowfat ice cream

Lunch

Chose ONE from column A and
Chose ONE from column B

<u>Column A</u>

1 cup lentil soup
1 cup pea soup
1 cup tomato soup or vegetable soup
1 cup bean with bacon soup
1 cup vegetable chili
½ cup vegetarian beans
½ cup nonfat refried beans
½ cup macaroni & cheese
1 cup pasta with tomato or primavera sauce
½ cup rice pudding
½ cup pudding made with skim milk
1 cup jello with nonfat whipped topping
1 cup nonfat frozen yogurt or low fat ice cream
1 apple
1 pear
1 orange
1 cup blueberries
1 cup raspberries

Skinny fruit cocktail
1 glass tomato juice
1 glass vegetable juice

Column B

1 pita bread or ½ bagel or 2 slices bread
     with ***Skinny Salad***
1 hamburger patty without the bun with lettuce,
     tomato and onion, or ***Skinny Salad***
1 individual can of water-packed tuna or chicken
     with ***Skinny Salad***
1 individual can sardines in water, olive oil, tomato
     or mustard sauce with ***Skinny Salad***
3 slices of nonfat ham, turkey or chicken
     with ***Skinny Salad***
3 slices of lowfat cheese with Skinny Salad
Skinny Omelet with ***Skinny Salad***
1 Tofu Burger with ***Skinny Salad***
4 ounces Vegetarian "meat substitute"
     with ***Skinny Salad***

Afternoon Snack Choices

Chose only ONE

3 pieces of celery with 1 tablespoon peanut butter
or 1 tablespoon low fat cheese spread
1 cup nonfat fruit yogurt
Skinny Sundae
Skinny Banana Split
1 cup nonfat frozen yogurt or low fat ice cream
1 apple
1 pear
1 orange
½ cantaloupe
1 cup strawberries
1 cup raspberries
1 cup blueberries
Skinny Fruit Salad
3 ounces of nonfat cheese

Dinner

Choose ONE From Column A and
Choose ONE From Column B and
Choose ONE From Column C

Column A

Skinny Salad with nonfat dressing
Sliced tomatoes and onions with nonfat dressing
Coleslaw made with nonfat dressing or mayo
Tossed green salad with nonfat dressing

Column B

Skinny Mixed Veggies
Skinny Steamed Veggies
Steamed asparagus
Steamed broccoli
Steamed cabbage
Steamed greens
Cooked beans
Cooked spinach
Steamed cauliflower
Cooked artichokes

Column C

8 ounces of skinless, boneless chicken, broiled, baked or grilled

8 ounces of skinless turkey, baked, broiled or grilled

8 ounces of lean steak, broiled or baked

1 hamburger patty, broiled or baked

8 ounces of fish, baked, broiled or grilled

Skinny Omelet

Tofu Burger

8 ounces Vegetarian "meat substitute"

Bedtime Snack

Chose ONE

Skinny Omelet
Skinny Deli Platter
1 cup nonfat fruit-flavored yogurt
3 ounces nonfat cheese
1 individual can water-packed tuna
 with *Skinny Salad*
1 individual can water-packed chicken
 with *Skinny Salad*
4 ounces Vegetarian "meat substitute"
 with *Skinny Salad*

Beverages

On *The Skinny Plan* you may unlimited quantities of the following beverages: water, club soda, decaf coffee, decaf tea, herbal tea.

You may have limited quantities of the following beverages: regular coffee, regular tea, diet soda, low fat soy beverage, low fat rice beverage. Please remember, try to limit your regular coffee, regular tea and diet soda to no more than 3 in a day in total. In other words do not exceed more than 3 cups of coffee, 3 cups of tea or 3 sodas in a day.

Acceptable Condiments

Mustard
Nonfat or reduced fat salad dressings
Nonfat mayo
Herbs & Spices
Horseradish
Ketchup (keep the ketchup to 1 tablespoon)

Salsa
Hot sauce
Salsa and hot sauce are hot calorie condiments and research says they may help boost your RMR and your fat burn. Use them generously.

RULE
All meats must be either baked, broiled or grilled. All fish must be either baked, broiled or grilled.

The 10 Minute Skinny Accelerator

What's so special about 10 minutes? How can 10-minutes fight my fat? Why a skinny accelerator? Because two different and independent studies showed that:

- 10 minute bouts of exercise increased compliance and reduced the risk of abandoning the exercise program.

- 10 minute bouts of exercise burned just as much fat and offered just as much cardiovascular benefit as longer workouts.

Now here is a new and remarkable study that combines the 10 minute concept with major Skinny benefits. I call it *The 10 Minute Skinny Accelerator.*

A study at Laval University in Canada found that intense exercise—in short bursts—burns off more body fat than less intense exercise.

Here's what the Laval University fat scientists did. They divided their study participants into two groups. They put each group on stationery bikes. What happened next can happen to you! Remember both groups pedaled for the same length of time. But it's the fat burn that is remarkable.

Group One	**Group Two**
Pedaled steadily	Pedaled in quick bursts
Burned more calories	Burned more fat— 9 times more fat!

You can give your body's own fat fighting chemistry a major boost with the 10 minute skinny accelerator. So just add a 10 minute skinny accelerator to your regular workout. If you walk, vary your pace and walk in bursts. If you bike, vary your pace and pedal in bursts. If you swim, vary your pace and swim faster for a couple of laps. The same skinny accelerator can be added to any workout. Just remember, vary your pace and "pump it up!"

Your Skinny Supporting Supplements

The Skinny Pill

Continue *The Skinny Pill* daily.

The same if you are using a do-it-yourself formula.

Calcium

Continue to take 2 calcium supplements daily. Each supplement should be at least 500 mg of calcium. Take one in the morning with water, orange juice, skim milk or a spoon or two of nonfat yogurt. Take the second at bedtime with water, skim milk, orange juice or a calcium-rich snack.

Antioxidant Supplement

Take at least one antioxidant supplement daily—two if you have checked with your doctor, pharmacist or other health care professional. Take each one with a full 8 ounces of water. When you are taking *The Skinny Pill*—mine or a do-it-yourself formula, it is a good idea to take your antioxidants at a different time—mid-afternoon or dinner are good choices.

Multivitamins

Take at least one multivitamin supplement daily—two if you have checked with your doctor, pharmacist or other health care professional. Take each one with a full 8 ounces of water. When you are taking *The Skinny Pill*, it is a good idea to take your multivitamins at a different time—mid-afternoon or dinner are good choices.

The Skinny Foods—Master Shopping List

Here is a master list of approved *Skinny Foods* that will help you keep winning your fat fight once you are ready to strike out on your own and put your own skinny meals together. But this is only if you have reached your skinny goal. If not, stay with the program.

Group 1

Angel food cake

Bagels

Bread, 7-grain

Bread, whole wheat

Bran cereal

Oatmeal

Muffins, bran low fat

Waffles, frozen

Pretzels

Crackers, whole grain

Tortillas, corn

Stuffing mix

Animal crackers

Bread, raisin

Bread, pita

Bread sticks

English muffins

Oat bran

Pancakes

Popcorn

Rice cakes

Sports bars

Breadcrumbs

Fig cookies

Group 2

Asparagus	Bok choy
Baked potatoes	Broccoli
Carrots	Cabbage
Cauliflower	Celery
Cucumbers	Peppers
Zucchini	Peas
Soybeans	Squash
Sweet potato	Pumpkin
Onion	Garlic
Scallions	Lettuce
Tomatoes	Dill

Group 3

Apples	Applesauce
Bananas	Apricots
Peaches	Pears
Oranges	Grapefruit
Fresh figs	Dates
Grapes	Cantaloupe
Pineapple	Strawberries
Raspberries	Blueberries
Raisins	Kiwi fruit
Assorted dried fruits	Papaya
Mango	Plums

Group 4

Skim milk
Cheeses, nonfat
Sour cream, nonfat

Yogurt, frozen,
Yogurt, nonfat

Group 5

Burritos, bean/beef
Egg substitutes
Tuna, water-packed
Refried beans, low fat
Chicken breasts
Steak
Veal
Halibut
Shellfish
Tofu burgers

Deli meat, low fat
Eggs
Nuts, dry roasted
Peanut butter
Turkey
Ground beef
Pork
Salmon, fresh
Salmon, canned
Vegetarian   Meat
Substitutes

Group 6

Coffee, regular & decaf
Tea, herbal & regular
Diet hot chocolate
Lowfat Rice Drink

Diet soda
Water
Lowfat Soy Drink

Part Six

Cooking Skinny

Sweet Treats

Oat Bran Balls

½ cup raisins
½ cup apple juice
1 cup oat bran
¼ cup nonfat dry milk powder
½ cup brown sugar

In a large bowl combine and mix all the ingredients. Add a little more juice if the mixture seems a little dry. Roll the dough into balls about the size of a small golf ball. Put into the fridge for about 15 minutes. Makes 2 dozen.

****
Give Your Kitchen A Make-Over
Throw out or donate all the foods that are making you fat and stock up on all the Skinny Foods that will help you win your fat fight.

Harvest Crisps

½ cup sugar
1 teaspoon cinnamon
½ teaspoon nutmeg
2 apples peeled, cored and sliced thin
24 graham crackers
8 ounces of cheddar cheese sliced, lowfat

Preheat oven to 350°F.

In a small bowl mix together the sugar, cinnamon, nutmeg and apples. Toss to coat well. Place the graham crackers on a nonstick cookie sheet. Evenly divide the coated apple slices, placing one on each cracker. Top with a small slice of and bake for 5 minutes until the cheese melts. Serve hot. Makes 24 servings.

****

A Little Fat Humor

"I have flabby thighs, but fortunately my stomach covers them." *Joan Rivers*.

Yes, You Can, Strawberry Shortcake

1 angel food cake
3 cups fresh strawberries, washed and sliced
1 tub (8 ounces) Cool Whip Free®, thawed

Cut cake into 6 generous slices. Reserve about 3 tablespoons of the strawberries. Place each slice on an individual dessert plate. Spoon about 3 tablespoons of the strawberries over and around the cake slices. Top each with about ¼ cup of the whipped topping. Garnish with a couple of slices of the remaining strawberries. Serve immediately. Makes 6 servings.

****
Take the Pencil Test

Can you keep a pencil tucked between your
"cheeks" and the tops of your thighs?
If it drops…you pass.
If it stays…you don't.

"I'm A Star" Fruit Cobbler

2 packages (16 ounces each) frozen sliced peaches
1 pint fresh blueberries
1 pint fresh raspberries
1 package (7 ounces) refrigerated buttermilk
      biscuits, low fat, separated
1 ¼ cups brown sugar
¼ cup cornstarch
1 pint nonfat vanilla frozen yogurt

Preheat oven to 475°F.

In a saucepan over medium heat combine the thawed peaches, blueberries, raspberries, sugar and cornstarch. Cook, stirring until thickened. Pour the mixture into a nonstick 12-inch x 8-inch baking dish. With a star-shaped cookie cutter, cut each biscuit into a star shape. Place the buttermilk biscuits over the fruit. Bake for 20 minutes or until the biscuit topping is lightly browned and the fruit is bubbling. Serve hot topped with a scoop of nonfat frozen vanilla yogurt. Makes 6 servings.

****
Smile
Those square meals? They can make you round!

Sweet Trifles

2 packages (3.4 ounces each) instant vanilla
     pudding mix
2 cups skim milk
2 cups sliced strawberries
2 cups blueberries
2 cups sliced kiwi fruit
24 vanilla wafers, broken into small pieces
½ cup strawberry all-fruit
1 cup nonfat whipped dairy topping

Prepare the pudding according to package instructions. In a separate bowl toss together the strawberries, blueberries and kiwi fruit. In individual parfait glasses arrange layers starting with a layer of cookies then berries, then pudding. Repeat. Chill for 30 minutes. Before serving top each glass with a generous scoop of whipped dairy topping.

****
Life's Little Chuckles

When choosing between two evils, I always like to try the one I've never tried before. *Mae West*

Savory Treats

Hearty Oven French Fries

3 medium baking potatoes, scrubbed but not
        peeled
½ teaspoon salt
1 tablespoon olive oil
¼ teaspoon ground black pepper
nonstick cooking spray

Preheat oven to 500°F

Spray two large cookie sheets with nonstick
cooking spray. Cut each potato lengthwise in half.
Put the cut side down and cutting lengthwise, slice
each half into ¼ inch slices. In a bowl, toss the
potatoes with the oil, salt and pepper. Divide the
coated potatoes evenly between the two cookie
sheets Bake 20 minutes or until brown. Turn the
potatoes with a spatula and bake another 5 to 10
minutes. Makes 4 servings.

****
Extra!
For a Mediterranean flavor add 1 teaspoon of dried
        oregano and 2 minced garlic cloves.

Salad Pizza

1 pizza crust, prepared according to package
1 cup shredded mozzarella, part skim
½ cup tomato sauce
2 cups romaine lettuce, shredded
1 tomato, chopped coarse
½ cup scallion, chopped coarse
4 cloves garlic, chopped fine
¼ cup low calorie Italian salad dressing
3 teaspoons grated parmesan cheese

Preheat oven to 500°F

Prepare pizza crust according to package directions and spread with tomato sauce and shredded mozzarella cheese. Bake for 5 minutes until the edges are golden. Remove from oven.

While pizza is baking in a large salad bowl toss together the lettuce, tomato, scallion, garlic, salad dressing and parmesan cheese. Load the salad onto the freshly baked pizza and enjoy. Makes 8 servings.

****
Laughter is inner jogging. *Norman Cousins*

Nachos Grande

4 cups baked tortilla chips
1 cup grated mozzarella cheese, low fat
¼ cup nonfat plain yogurt
¼ cup nonfat sour cream
1 cup canned green chilis, minced

Preheat broiler.

Arrange tortilla chips on a nonstick cookie sheet. In a bowl combine the mozzarella cheese, yogurt, sour cream and chilis. Spoon the mixture over the tortilla chips. Broil until bubbling. Serve hot. Serves 6.

****

Getting "The Blues" May Help You Lose The Fat

Researchers at Johns Hopkins found that hot colors
like red and orange crank up your appetite.
Cool colors like blue or green turn it down.
So get out that paint brush and "cool down" your
kitchen and dining room!

Smoked Salmon Bites

4 ounces smoked salmon cut into strips
¾ cup nonfat ricotta cheese
¼ cup nonfat cream cheese
1 teaspoon lemon juice

In your food processor combine all ingredients. Blend until mixture is smooth. Serve with raw veggies, slices of toasted bagel, or crackers.
Makes 4 servings.

****
Think About This One

It's a funny thing about life;
if you refuse to accept anything
but the best, you very often get it.
Somerset Maugham

Three-Bean Salad

1 16-ounce can cut green beans, drained
1 16-ounce can yellow wax beans, drained
1 16-ounce can kidney beans, drained
1 small green pepper, seeded and chopped fine
1 small red pepper, seeded and chopped fine
1 small onion, peeled and chopped fine
½ cup nonfat Italian salad dressing

Combine all ingredients in a large glass salad bowl. Chill until ready to serve. Makes 12 servings.

****
Who's Winning The Fat Wars?
Women.

All American Comfort Foods

TexMex Chips

8 5 ½-inch corn tortillas
¼ teaspoon ground cumin
¼ teaspoon ground coriander
¼ teaspoon chili powder
¼ teaspoon salt
nonstick cooking spray

Preheat oven to 350°F.

In a bowl combine the cumin, coriander, chile powder and salt. Spray both sides of the tortillas with cooking spray and sprinkle with the spice mixture. Cut each tortilla into 6 wedges. Arrange on a nonstick cookie sheet and bake 15 to 18 minutes or until crisp. Serve slightly warm with your favorite salsa. Makes 8 servings.

****
National Institutes of Health Guidelines
Live healthier
Exercise
Change your diet to reduce fat
Think thin. Think positive

Savory & Sweet Potato Wedges

2 sweet potatoes, peeled and sliced lengthwise
      into 6 wedges
1 teaspoon olive oil
½ teaspoon curry powder
¼ teaspoon ground cumin
¼ teaspoon ground cinnamon
¼ teaspoon salt
¼ teaspoon pepper

Preheat oven to 425°F.

In a large bowl toss the potato wedges with the oil and spices until evenly coated. Place the coated wedges on a nonstick cookie sheet. Bake for 20 to 30 minutes until tender. Makes 4 servings.

****
Words of Wisdom
If you want your dreams to come true…
Don't sleep.

Man, That's Great Chili

1 pound ground turkey, or lean ground sirloin
1 large onion, peeled and chopped
2 24-ounce cans seasoned stewed tomatoes
1 large green pepper, seeded and chopped
1 large red pepper, seeded and chopped
1 small can green chilis, chopped
1 16-ounce can tomato sauce
2 16-ounce cans seasoned chili beans
1 cup brown rice, uncooked
2 tablespoons chili powder
1 teaspoon garlic powder
dash of pepper to taste
vegetable cooking spray

In a large stockpot brown the turkey and onion in a little of the vegetable cooking spray. Add all the remaining ingredients. Bring to a boil. Reduce heat and simmer for 1 hour. Pour into bowls. Serve with saltine crackers. Makes 12 servings.

****

What is America's favorite day to start a diet?
Monday is the winner.

Brunswick Stew

1 tablespoon vegetable oil
1 medium onion, peeled and chopped
1 pound boneless, skinless chicken breasts
          cut into cubes
1 14 ½-ounce can seasoned, stewed tomatoes,
          chopped coarse
1 6-ounce can tomato paste
1 10-ounce package frozen lima beans
1 10-ounce package frozen corn kernels
1 10 ½-ounce can chicken stock
1 10 ½-ounce can water
2 tablespoons Worcestershire sauce
1 teaspoon lemon juice
dash of hot pepper sauce

In a deep skillet heat the oil over medium-high heat. Add the onion and chicken breast. Brown lightly. Add the remaining ingredients. Bring to a boil. Reduce heat and simmer covered for 1 hour. Makes 6 servings.

Baked Beans

1 tablespoon vegetable oil
3 cloves garlic, peeled and minced
2 small onions, peeled and chopped fine
2 teaspoons dried mustard
5 cups cooked navy beans
3 tablespoons honey
dash of hot pepper sauce to taste

Preheat oven to 325°. In an oven-safe pot on top of the stove heat the oil at medium-high heat. Add the garlic, onions and mustard until the onions are lightly golden. Add all the remaining ingredients. Mix together. Cover and bake for 3 hours stirring from time to time. Makes 6 servings.

****
Did You Know?
The average weight of men in their forties
is 173 pounds compared with 140 pounds
100 years ago!

Part Seven

Resources

Most Often Asked Questions

Will I get skinny if I just take *The Skinny Pill* and don't follow *The Skinny Food Clock*?
You might. Or you might not. The point is that this program is not just about taking a pill and continuing poor, unhealthy eating habits.

If I decide to put together my own formula will I get the same results?
Because I can't guarantee the potency or bioavailability of other products or ingredients I can't tell you that you will get the same result.

How much will I lose on *The Skinny Pill*?
Everyone is different. But many people who have already been on the program have lost up to one pound a day for five days and continue to lose up to 21 pounds in the first month. People lose at approximately twice the rate they would normally.

How will I feel?
You should begin to feel energized within the first 24 hours after starting. You should also feel a real difference in the consistency of your fat. It will feel less like Silly Putty and more like Jello.

What if I go off *The Skinny Pill*?

What happens when you go off any health modification program?

I don't like some of the food that you list in your daily menus. Can I make substitutions?

For the first 30 days I prefer you to stick to *The Skinny Pill* and *The Skinny Food Clock* just as written.

Can I mix and match the meals?

You may switch breakfast for breakfast, lunch for lunch, dinner for dinner and so on. If you are in a bind and can't eat the suggested foods for a given day, just look on the list of do-it-yourself substitutes and pick your meals from that extensive list of skinny breakfasts, lunches, dinners and snacks.

I'm a vegetarian.

The basics to remember are eat your fibers and carbs before noon and your proteins after noon. I also recommend that you substitute fish for the meat choices or omelets. You can also select from the variety of vegetarian foods in my do-it-yourself list.

Selected References

Better Nutrition. February 1996. January 1995. September 1994.

Campbell, W., Beard, J.L., Joseph, L., et al. 1997. *American Journal of Clinical Nutrition.*

Clancy, S.P., Clarkson, P.M., DeCheke, M.E., et al. 1994. *International Journal of Sport Nutrition.*

Colombani, R., Wenk, C., Kuntz, I., et al. 1996. *European Journal of Applied Physiology.*

Gormley, J., *Better Nutrition.* May 1996. March 1997.

Grant, K.E. *Medicine and Science in Sports and Exercise.* 1997.

Harper, P., Wadstrom, C., et al. 1995. *American Journal of Clinical Nutrition.*

Jaros, T. *Vegetarian Times.* February 1996.

Kalman, D. S., *Muscular Development.* July, 1998.

Murray, F. *Better Nutrition.* 1992.

Nielsen, F.H. *Nutrition Today.* 1996.

Nutrition Health Review. Spring. 1993.

Press, R.I., Geller, J., and Evans, G. *Western Journal of Medicine.* 1990.

Reading, S. A. *Journal of the Florida Medical Association.* 1996.

Rowley, B. 1997. *Muscle and Fitness.*

Trent, L.K., and Thielding-Cancel, D. *Journal of Sports Medicine and Physical Fitness.* 1995.

Tufts University Diet & Nutrition Letter. October 1996. January 1997.

Watanbe, S., Ajisaka, R., Masuoka, R., et al. 1995. *Japanese Heart Journal.*

Do-It-Yourself Skinny Pill

All the components for *The Skinny Pill* formula which you can assemble yourself are readily available at most outlets that sell herbal products and vitamins. Here is the formula to put together for yourself:

L'carnitine	250 mg
Chromium	400 mcg
Citrimax	300 mg
Chitosan	250 mg
Citrus Aurantium	300 mg

Supporting Skinny Supplements

Vitamin C	200 to 1,000 mg
Beta-carotene	50 to 10,000 IU
Vitamin E	30 to 800 IU
Calcium	1,000 to 1,500 mg

How To Order Edita's *Skinny Pill*

30-DAY SUPPLY SKINNY PILL $29.99

SPECIAL! $59.98
Order 2 months get ONE MONTH FREE!

Please add $5.95 S&H to all orders.
Florida residents add 6% sales tax.
Allow 2 to 4 weeks for delivery.

Make checks or money orders payable to:
The Skinny Pill
830-13 Route A1A North
Ponte Vedra Beach, FL 32082

Toll Free Order Numbers:
1-800-870-8087 or 1-888-7-Skinny

Shop On Line
www.theskinnypill.com

Most major credit cards accepted.
All Sales Final. No Returns.